LISTEN TO WHAT THE STARS AND THE PRESS SAY ABOUT MICHAEL MARON'S INSTANT MAKEOVER MAGIC

"A self-improvement manual with a difference. His book not only informs and instructs but . . . carries an aura of genuine concern and artistic integrity . . . interesting reading, entertaining as well as informative."
—*San Diego Magazine*

"Women will find this manual most useful for Maron's concrete tips on accentuating good features and minimizing others . . . this volume demonstrates that with a little thought and effort, a lot can be done to glamorize one's image."
—*Publisher's Weekly*

"Excellent advice. . . . It is startling to see women we've always seen as glamorous and beautiful in their 'natural' state. And it is even more startling to see what the right makeup can do for anyone—famous or not."
—*Big Beautiful Woman*

"Some of the greatest before and after shots ever assembled . . . an especially appealing aspect of the book is the inclusion of makeover subjects of all ages and figure styles."
—*San Jose Mercury News*

"Michael has made me feel like a classic beauty. His makeup and work is indeed 'magic.' I am pleased to be part of it."
—Mariette Hartley

"Michael's sensitivity as an artist adds up to sheer genius."
—Lynda Carter

"He's a fantastic talent. Look what he did with me! Now that I know I can be a sex symbol, I'll never be the same, thanks to the fantastic talents of Michael Maron."
—Ruth Buzzi

"I love Michael's work so much! I'm just amazed and very proud."
—Nastassia Kinski

"I thank you from the bottom of my heart for your time and talent."
—Linda Gray

"I'm sure everyone will learn from and love this book." —Donna Pescow

"What a delight to be in Michael's book . . . that Maron touch of genius will make it a keepsake." —Cyd Charisse

"One leaves a session with Michael looking and feeling beautiful." —Juliet Prowse

"He has won me. From now on I will consider him 'the best.'" —Morgan Brittany

"Michael applies his makeup so naturally that you look like a natural beauty." —Cheryl Ladd

"This year's most enlightening, enchanting and thoroughly helpful 'how to' book." —*Drama-Logue*, Los Angeles

MICHAEL MARON'S INSTANT MAKEOVER MAGIC

MICHAEL MARON

Introduction by Carol Burnett

Photographs by Michael Maron

WARNER BOOKS

A Warner Communications Company

Warner Books Edition

Copyright © 1983 by Michael P. Maron

This Warner Books edition is published by arrangement with
Rawson Associates, 597 Fifth Avenue, New York, NY 10107

Warner Books, Inc., 666 Fifth Avenue, New York, NY 10103
(W) A Warner Communications Company

Printed in the United States of America

First Warner Books Printing: February 1985

10   9   8   7   6   5

Front cover photograph and photograph on page 13 of Michael Maron
© 1984 by Harry Langdon Photography

Library of Congress Cataloging in Publication Data

Maron, Michael.
    Michael Maron's instant makeover magic.

    Reprint. Originally published: New York:
Rawson Associates, 1983.
    Includes index.
    1. Beauty, Personal.   2. Cosmetics.   3. Hair—Care
and hygiene.   4. Clothing and dress.   I. Title.
[RA778.M355   1985]   646.7'042   84-17276
ISBN   0-446-38187-X(U.S.A.)(pbk.)
    0-446-38188-8(Canada)(pbk.)

To the most beautiful woman I know —
my mother, Della. I love you, Mom.

CONTENTS

INTRODUCTION

BY CAROL BURNETT

When my friend Bob Mackie first told me of Michael Maron's project, I was flattered that Michael wanted me to be in the book. When Michael told me that most of the women would be photographed without any makeup at all, I asked him who would be writing the introduction, Vincent Price?

I assume Mr. Price was not available.

Michael explained that he wanted to use before as well as after photographs to show that every woman has her own unique look—and that the magic is in learning how to recognize one's best features.

I became interested in Michael's talents because I've always believed in growth and change. As you can see from his photos, he complements his subjects' best features with the application of ten easy makeup steps, combining the art of makeup and photography for impressive results.

I've never considered myself one of the world's most sought-after women by authors of beauty books, so I'm doubly pleased to be in the company of all the women presented in these pages. You will see different types of women, just like you and me, some of whom are not the faces you'd expect to see.

Michael's approach is based on the feeling that beauty is a matter of feeling good about one's self, liking one's self, and doing whatever is necessary to enhance those feelings. His book shows, simply, how to achieve these goals inside and out.

I know you'll enjoy this book as much as I have enjoyed being part of it.

Carol Burnett

ACKNOWLEDGMENTS

I'd like to thank all of the beautiful women photographed here who chose to share themselves with us in order to have us see them in a way many of them have never been seen by the public before. That is to say, without any makeup at all. Because of the use of the word *makeover* in connection with this book, I'd like to make it clear that I'm not implying that I created the images by which we have come to recognize them. But I particularly chose a number of well-known, recognizable personalities in order to illustrate the point that almost everyone, beginning with their own natural "naked" face, can create a particular image when correct makeup is applied to further enhance their own special uniqueness and natural assets.

As we know, the ability to project the full range of human expression is inherent in each of us. Therefore, the look you might choose for yourself should be the one that you are most comfortable with and which works to accommodate a variety of moods and roles. Labels aren't important; your own uniqueness is.

I wish to express my gratitude to all these women and to the personal managers, secretaries, publicists, agents, and friends, whose wonderful cooperation and support resulted in the book you have before you. Particularly in a business that can sometimes base the potential success of one's career on image and appearance, I find it courageous and especially loving of these women to have volunteered to show a personal revelation to a public which most often sees *only* the stereotypical image. I believe this shows a sense of confidence and a depth of character. I cannot minimize the importance of this sharing and giving. I also want to thank the many doctors, skin care experts, nutritionists, health and physical fitness authorities, clothing designers, and fashion consultants who contributed their time and efforts so graciously. Special thanks go to the many talented hair stylists with whom I work for their beautiful contributions to makeover magic.

I am especially indebted to Michael Chapman, my inspiration and best friend, for his artistic guidance and creative input and for his sincere devotion, laughter, and loving support.

I gratefully acknowledge the talents of Paddy Calistro McAuley and her thoughtfulness and skill in helping me prepare this book.

Special thanks to Suzanne Stanford for her support and dedication and for coordinating the myriad details necessary to the photographic contributions of the women in this book.

I'd like to thank Eleanor and Ken Rawson, my publishers, for knowing a good thing when they saw it and for lending their special expertise to the final results. Thanks, too, to Sandra Choron for knowing how to make a good thing look its best.

For the many hours of excellent work at Lens-Art Photo Lab, I wish to thank Shirley Borchardt, Harold Goodfried, Chang Pak, Eny Sohn, and Ferenc Tiszai.

For always believing in me and for buying me my first camera, I thank my father, Joseph Maron. Thanks, Dad!

Thanks to Elizabeth Backman, my agent, and to all my dear friends for their constant enthusiasm and love. Thank you: Larry Austin, Julian Ayrs, Roslyn Baws, J. Edgar Bledsoe, John Bowab, David Funt, Jacqueline Green, Michelle Hart, Ole Henriksen, Marti Hopps, Eric Stephen Jacobs, Eric Lasher, Maureen Lasher, Barbara Lauren, Liz Marshall, James Maxwell, Ivana Moore, Roberta Nooger, Marvin Paige, Carol Paradis, Vivian Polak, Andrea Sells, Esther Spencer, Judy Varon, Timothy Wayne, Jeffrey Wernick.

1

PUTTING YOUR BEST FACE FORWARD

When Carol Burnett walked into my photo studio on a rainy March afternoon, it was as if the sun had come out from behind the clouds. The room lit up. She's one of the most spirited and enthusiastic people I've ever met, and at the same time, she's slightly shy and soft-spoken. It's immediately obvious why she's one of the best-loved women in America. She radiates an inner beauty—a charismatic warmth—that's matched by her fabulous smile, her beautiful eyes, and those great legs. When I first saw her in her jeans and a T-shirt, she came across like so many women who don't realize how pretty they really are. When I asked her if she felt as gorgeous as she looked, she blushed

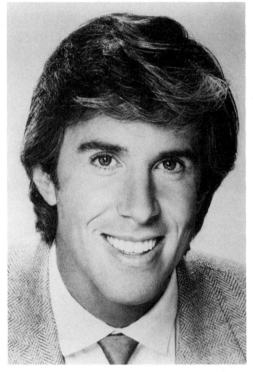

and poked fun at herself: "If you want to shoot my best side, can you shoot the back of my head?"

If you think you have nothing in common with Carol or with Lynn Redgrave, Nastassia Kinski, Lynda Carter, Cyd Charisse, Cheryl Ladd, or any of the other beautiful women in this book, I'm going to prove that you're mistaken. They're women just like you, who wake up in the morning and occasionally focus on a blemish here, a wrinkle there, a nose they may think is too big (or too small), a chin that recedes (or juts too much)—or whatever. And they forget to look at that gorgeous smile, those beautiful eyes, a wonderful head of hair, or a face full of unique features that add up to a very special whole.

That's not so unusual. Most of us can't look at ourselves objectively. We're constantly measuring our looks by images we see on TV, in magazines, or on the movie screen.

Everyone has something about themselves that they'd like to change; it's human nature. But I'm here to tell you—a thousand times, if necessary—that you are beautiful *now*! Don't ever try to look like someone else. I want to show you how to maximize *your* assets. I'll show you, in ten very easy steps, how to apply makeup to enhance your features. I'll explain how changing a hair style can create a fresh new look. And I'll teach you how to carefully evaluate your figure and your wardrobe so you can dress to suit your new image. These are the three phases to my makeover magic: makeup, hair, and image. You just have to be willing to allow yourself the pleasure of looking wonderful.

In this book, you'll find photographs of many women, celebrities and others who may be less familiar to you. But I assure you that rarely does anyone roll out of bed looking like the "after" photographs you're about to enjoy. The results you see in these photos are based on the concepts I want to share with you—correct makeup application, choosing the right hair style, wearing the right clothes to suit your face and figure, good skin care, planning a successful health and fitness program, building self-confidence, and selecting the professionals who can help you if you need it.

Each of us has a special uniqueness—an inner beauty that surfaces no matter what. Whenever I work with people, I always try to bring that out. The thrill I get every time I see someone feel better about themselves by putting her or his best face forward makes me love what I do.

As a portrait painter and photographer, I learned what color, shading, and light can do to create a natural-looking beautiful face. I found that with makeup, I could use the same concepts of light and dark on a face that I had used on canvas. Now, as a makeup artist, I can *instantly* turn an ordinary face into a dazzling face. To me, this is magic!

As a beauty, fashion, and personality photographer and makeup artist, I am faced daily with the joy of helping to create exciting images for my clients. Having worked in front of the camera as an actor also has helped me to understand how one's appearance affects others.

When clients first enter my studio, we sit down and talk—to relax, to get to know a little more about each other, and to allow me time to study their faces. I watch their eyes. I look at their expressions. I analyze their bone structure. I look at their skin, hair, teeth, eyebrows. I listen to what they say about the way they live. These are important things that add up to the image I want my camera to capture.

Carol Burnett made this phase of our session easy. She was so honest and open about herself that it was simple to capture her own natural warmth and beauty. "I don't feel extremely confident putting on my own makeup, even though I can do it fairly well," Carol admitted. "I'm a very good student. If someone tells me where it goes, I can do it; but if I have to figure it out myself, I'm lost. If the steps are too complicated, I'll do it once or twice and forget it. As far as skin care goes, I wash my face with whatever soap I have around. I use a moisturizer if I remember, and that's it—no facials, no magic potions. I spend a great deal of time in the sun, even though I know it's bad for my skin. I wear a strong sun block with a sun protection factor of 15 under my eyes, but I like to get color, so I wear a weaker strength (SPF 4 or 6) on the rest of my face. In the daytime I like to look very natural, but sometimes I really enjoy looking glamorous at night. My friend, designer Bob Mackie, has made some fabulous beaded sheaths that make me feel very glamorous. It's such a different image. My audiences never think of me as beautiful or glamorous. I remind them of their sister or their niece or their daughter. There's an amateurishness about me that people relate to."

As we chatted in my makeup room, I continued analyzing Carol's features: huge blue eyes, a clear complexion, an even skin tone, a great smile, beautiful teeth, and a straight nose. Then we began the makeover process.

I used a little concealer to erase the dark areas at the inner corners of her eyes and applied highlighter above her cheekbones and on the sides of her face directly below the contour area to create a wider illusion for her narrow face. Although she had always thought her large mouth a liability, I told her it was one of her best features and accentuated her lips with coral lipstick. I even made her lips look a bit wider by using a reddish brown lip liner outside her natural lip line. A frosted pink lipstick in the center of her lower lip and a bit of gloss made her look sexy without looking too made up. Carol was delighted to see herself looking natural *and* glamorous at the same time.

We didn't have to change her hair one bit. After eleven years as the

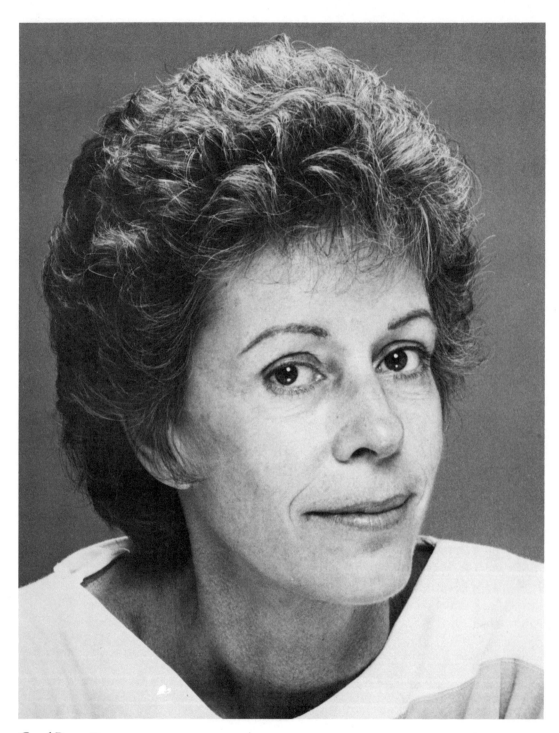

Carol Burnett

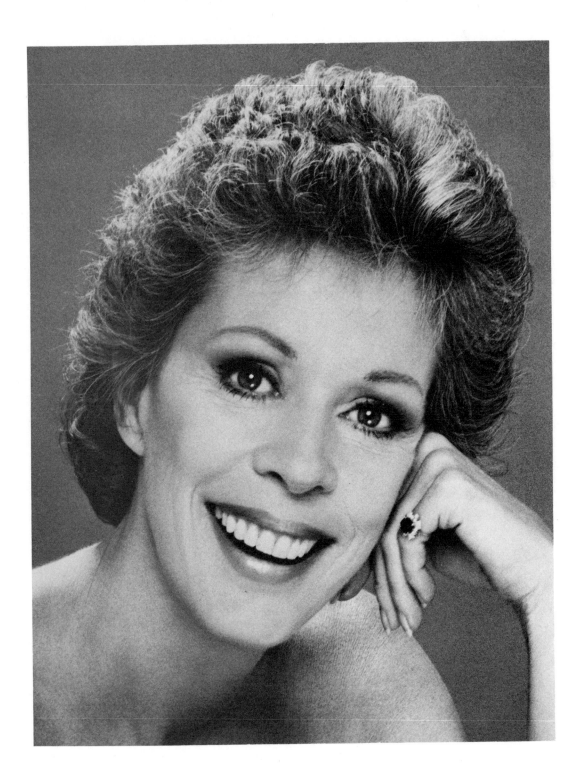

redheaded star of her own show, Carol had let her hair grow out to its natural light brown, now liberally sprinkled with glistening threads of gray. Her colorist, Virginia, of Vidal Sassoon in Beverly Hills, added a few touches of golden blond. "For years I did my color myself, and I guess that's why it was never the same for two months in a row. I just bought a bottle of red and used it—any brand, I wasn't particularly discriminating. When the show was over, I was ready to go back to my natural shade." Her short cut with fullness at the top and sides is the perfect frame for her long, narrow face. "It's so easy. I get a perm every three or four months and it always looks like this. I get an occasional trim—no regular pattern, just whenever I need it."

In this book you will see women the way I see them—before and after. The photographs I've presented are intended to illustrate the magical differences a little makeup, a fresh hairstyle, a new neckline, or a different attitude can make in your overall appearance. As you turn the pages, you're likely to find a woman who has the same face shape as yours and another with the same nose or maybe the same hair or figure problem. You'll see how I deal with their features, and then you can try the same techniques yourself. There are no long, difficult procedures. Because the truth of the matter is that with a touch of blusher here, a trace of shadow there, and perhaps a simple new hairstyle, any woman can look dazzling—in minutes. And none of my makeup techniques are too complicated to do in front of your own mirror. The women I've worked with tell me they're easily able to follow my ten easy makeup steps and achieve the same wonderful results on their own.

The art of photography is very exacting and tends to capture, in a moment of time, shadings and lines that the human eye doesn't see. Occasionally I have employed the techique of retouching, but there is no retouching on the "after" shots that doesn't also appear on the "befores." Any retouching of photographs used in these pages is to correct photographic flaws only, *not to alter the effects of a makeover*. Furthermore, I always used identical lighting techniques on both shots. I'm not here to mislead you.

I have chosen to use black and white photographs rather than color for a very specific reason. Black and white makes it easier to see form, placement, and shading. Color photographs reproduced in books and magazines often suffer in the printing process and can look different from the original image. Often this difference is both misleading and confusing when the subject is makeup.

All phases of the makeover process will be discussed in the pages that follow just as I explain them to my clients. And as I always emphasize, we're going to *enhance* you, not *change* you.

First, I'll go into detail about each step in the makeup process to show you precisely how to apply cosmetics for a natural, fresh-faced look. I'll also show you several before and after photos of women so you can see exactly how each step plays an important part in their final look.

Then we'll tackle the second phase of your makeover—your hair. I've selected a number of before and after photos that demonstrate how simple hair changes can often make startling differences.

To complete the makeover process, we'll deal with your total image. We'll focus on your clothes, your posture, your attitude, and what I like to call inner beauty. Fashion designers will offer tips on buying clothes. The accompanying makeover photos will show you how a simple change can positively enhance your figure, and a number of women will tell how their new look has made them feel great about themselves.

We'll also briefly discuss those optional changes such as corrective dentistry, electrolysis, cosmetic surgery. These are the changes you can make if you have the time, money, and inclination. I always encourage my clients to make any changes that make them feel better. Years ago women—especially celebrities—didn't want to talk about the diets they went on or the facelifts they'd had. Now many stars are more open about the positive changes they've made in their appearance.

Without my asking, Carol Burnett told me all about her recent corrective surgery. After years of dissatisfaction with her profile, she finally decided to do something about her chin. "I heard about a form of oral surgery that could alter the line of my jaw, so I looked into it. I learned that the operation could be done in an hour, under general anesthesia. My oral surgeon showed me X-rays and diagrams and demonstrated exactly what kind of changes could be made. The procedure brought my jaw forward about four millimeters. That's a very tiny change, yet it made a difference in how I felt when I looked in the mirror. After all these years I have a chin."

And even Carol—yes, model-thin, five-foot-six-and-three-quarter-inch, 112-pound Carol with those fabulous legs—admits to having had a weight problem. She credits her svelte body to eating slowly, taking small portions, and having the discipline to stop after one or two bites of dessert. "I'm not a martyr," she laughs. "I don't deprive myself, but I don't overindulge, either. After I had my third daughter, I was up to one hundred and forty pounds and a size fourteen. Bob Mackie teased me a little, but I really didn't think the problem was serious until a woman in the audience asked me when my next baby was due—and I *wasn't* pregnant! I went on a diet immediately and got down to a hundred and twenty-five, which was a big improvement. Gradually, I lost the rest, and I feel like I'm finally at the right weight. Actually, I don't care if I weigh three hundred pounds, as long as I can fit into a size seven. I buy tight jeans, and if they get tighter I watch what I eat." I will show you before and after photos of women like Carol who wanted to make some permanent changes and did—with wonderful results.

Throughout this book, you'll meet many of your favorite celebrities. They're women who know a great deal about beauty and want to share some of their personal knowledge with you. It is my hope that their secrets, along with my own program, will bring you the joy and satisfaction that my clients and friends experience.

2

TEN STEPS
TO INSTANT
MAKEOVER MAGIC

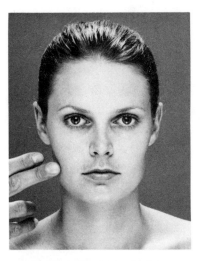
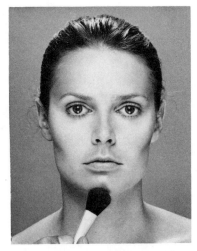
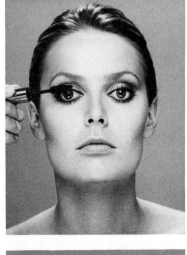
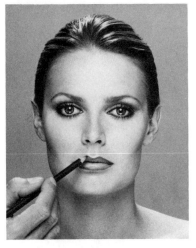
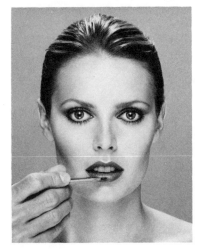
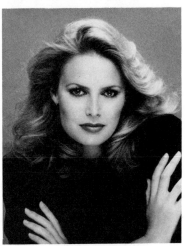

*I*t might seem that transforming a face from nice to knockout would be a difficult process—but it isn't. In fact, as you'll see in the next few pages, it's done in ten easy steps. Although many different cosmetics may be used in my makeovers, careful blending and a light-handed touch will produce a soft, natural-looking face. Even when you're doing a glamorous, sophisticated makeup for a special night out, you still should look as natural as possible. For these dramatic evenings, you'll simply use more intense colors, again blending to create the most natural look possible. Correct application is more important than color or intensity.

Every face is inherently beautiful. Often I've found that playing up the very things that you may hope to minimize is the secret to a beautiful face. Don't make yourself crazy trying to figure out whether you have a round, square, oval, oblong, or heart-shaped face—most faces are a combination of shapes. You have *your* face, and together we're going to enhance it.

Now, on with the process! Naturally, you'll need some tools, most of which you probably have on hand or which are available at your local beauty supply or drug store. Here's what you'll need:

- 2 large fluffy, sable-hair brushes (approximately 1 inch wide)
- 3 small sable-hair brushes (approximately 1/4 inch wide)
- 1 square-tipped lip brush
- 1 eyebrow brush or child's toothbrush
- 1 eyelash curler
- Cotton swabs
- Latex sponges
- Cotton balls
- A hand mirror

These are the essentials. Good quality brushes are a must. Most of the cosmetic brush kits available will include these sizes and a few extras. I like the short-handled versions because they travel well, but select whatever style you prefer as long as the brushes are sable. There are a variety of excellent kits available at many department and beauty supply stores. A less expensive alternative is to visit an art supply store, where you'll find a large selection of sable brushes. It's very important to wash the brushes frequently in mild soap and water, since used brushes can breed bacteria. Use a hair dryer at medium heat to dry them quickly. Beauty supply stores also carry instant-drying cleaning solvents for brushes, if you prefer that.

I use latex sponges to apply foundation. They don't absorb too much color, which allows for a light, even application without streaking. It's important to rinse your sponge after each use so it doesn't harbor germs. Since I work with so many different faces, I use a fresh sponge for each foundation application. I buy sponges in bulk and then cut each one into sixths, angling off one end to form a wedge. Precut sponges are available in stores but cost about twice the price. If you can't find cosmetic grade latex sponges, write to Frends Beauty Supply Company, the largest supplier of theatrical makeup in Hollywood, at 5202 Laurel Canyon Boulevard, North Hollywood, California 91607.

The light surrounding your mirror will make a big difference in the way your makeup looks. Always try to apply makeup in the same kind of light in which you'll be seen. For the most natural condition, place your mirror between two windows so that both sides of your face are equally lit. Incandescent light—yes, the kind you get from ordinary bulbs—is the next best thing to natural light. Avoid overhead lighting, which casts odd shadows. Fluorescent light, which you find in most offices, can be very harsh and cast extremely unflattering shadows. Many portable makeup mirrors have a setting that simulates fluorescent lighting so that you see how your makeup will look under these conditions. (You may find that you want to use a bit more pink in your cosmetics to soften the effect of those glaring lights.) Use your hand mirror to help check makeup from all angles.

A special note to contact lens wearers: I've seen gorgeous eye makeup ruined by the insertion of a wet lens. Chances are you'll do a much better job on your eyes if you wear your lenses while you apply your makeup. Just be particularly careful not to get particles of makeup in your eyes.

Another tool you'll need is one you probably owned as a teenager but haven't used since: an eyelash curler. It's one of the most important tools. Even long-lashed lovelies like Linda Gray and Nastassia Kinski benefit from using this clever little contraption. It lifts the lashes to make them seem longer and makes the eyes look larger. The standard Maybelline and Kurlash curlers, sold in drug or variety stores, work very well. Jonee makes a deluxe curler called Excellence, which I use in my work. It has a quick spring action and carries its own piggyback supply of extra rubber strips. You can get one by writing Jonee Inc., 9034 Bermudez, Pico Rivera, California 90660. Whichever type you choose, make sure to replace the little rubber strip frequently, since it can pull out lashes if it's worn.

Underneath It All—Cleansing Your Skin

Virginia Mayo has learned the importance of good skin care. She removes all makeup with Albolene cream, washes thoroughly with Ivory or pure castile soap, and rinses with warm water. She wears a light moisturizer underneath her foundation.

So many of my clients who have beautiful skin tell me that they only wear makeup when they work, that they like to let their skin "breathe" after hours. Of course, the skin doesn't "breathe," whether you're wearing makeup or not, but what these women are saying is what skin care expert Georgette Klinger expressed to me so well: "The face must be naked some of the time."

Many skin specialists believe that wearing makeup all the time clogs the pores and causes blemishes or enlarged pores. There's another school of skin care, however, which claims that makeup, especially foundation, protects the skin from the elements. You'll have to be the judge. If your skin responds well to a day off from cosmetics, do it regularly. If you have clear skin and wear makeup all the time, no need to change. In either case, be sure to cleanse your skin well at least twice a day, especially before bed.

First, remove your eye makeup with an oily product designed to dissolve the mascara, powders, pencils, and creams you've applied to the eye area. I recommend unscented Albolene cream as an effective and inexpensive makeup remover. The eye area is very delicate, so treat it lovingly. Never pull or stretch the skin. Use cotton balls to gently wipe away the remains of the day's eye makeup. Never use cheap facial tissue to remove your makeup; the wood fibers in it can damage your skin.

Then, using a cleansing lotion, gently remove the rest of the makeup from your face and neck. Using upward, outward, circular motions, gently massage the lotion into your face for one minute. As the makeup dissolves, wipe away the residue with a damp cotton ball or washcloth. Splash your face several times with warm (not hot) water until all the makeup is gone.

Now, using a mild soap (you'll find several kinds at health food stores; I prefer the unscented brands) and a clean terry washcloth, gently massage your skin again to clean your pores and exfoliate the dead skin cells that have accumulated during the day. Most people have combination skin with oily patches on the nose and forehead, so massage these areas carefully to remove the built-up film. Rinse again with tepid water. Blot your face gently with your softest, most luxurious towel. Go over your face with a cotton ball moistened with freshener or toner to further remove any residue. A spritz of mineral water adds an extra touch of moisture to your skin.

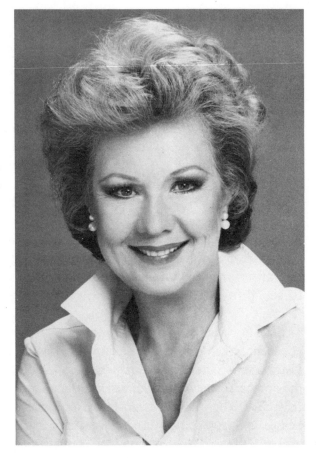

Virginia Mayo
(Hairstyle by Eric Root)

The next step is moisturizer. Despite its name, a moisturizer does not moisturize your skin. It seals in the moisture that only water can provide. Dry skin results when your skin loses its natural moisture. If you have dry skin, immediately after using freshener or toner and mineral water, apply a rich, greaseless moisturizer to seal in this surface moisture.

It isn't always necessary to use expensive skin care products. The noted dermatologist Dr. Arnold Klein says that "Vaseline petroleum jelly is the best moisturizer you can buy, but most people hate to use such a heavy ointment." He also says that people with dry skin should not use soap and water and recommends Cetaphil lotion as an effective dry skin cleanser. As a matter of fact, Dr. Klein complains that more damage is done to the skin by overcleaning it than by almost anything else (except the sun). "Americans are convinced that their skin is dirty," he asserts. "Acne, for instance, has nothing to do with dirt—it's a hormonal problem."

If your skin is only slighty dry to normal, you can get away with a light moisturizer or with one of the oil-free moisturizing products. If you have oily skin, you don't need any extra oils that might clog your pores overnight.

The area around the eyes has no oil glands. Special eye creams, which are rich with emollients, help keep this delicate region supple, reducing the chances of fine lines. Start using eye cream now, before it's too late.

There are longer, more expensive regimens for a healthy complexion, but as I've said, my aim is to keep things simple. I *can* promise that if you follow this very simple routine at bedtime every night, you're on your way to better, more beautiful skin.

According to Hollywood's skin care expert Ole Henriksen, your skin relaxes and recovers from the stresses of the day as you sleep in the same way the rest of your body does. Your clean skin will naturally excrete excess oils and pollutants, and new cells will continue to develop, forcing old cells to die and sit on the surface of your skin. This is your skin's natural rejuvenation process. Be sure that you allow enough time for this process to take place; get enough sleep.

And because your skin has undergone this healthy transformation while you slept, it's imperative that you wash your face first thing in the morning. Using a superfatted soap and a terry washcloth, wash your face, sloughing off the dead cells and washing away the pollutants and oils your skin has expelled. If you're going to need a sun block during the day, smooth it on your face before you apply moisturizer or makeup. I always recommend sunblock lotions with an SPF (sun protection factor) of 15, since those products best shield your skin from the harmful rays of the sun.

Smoking prematurely ages your skin. It not only causes the vessels in the eyes to constrict but can affect the color of your skin and cause the formation of tiny, aging lines. A word to the wise . . .

Grocery Store Facials

Sometimes your skin needs a little extra attention. You can treat yourself to a professional facial if you're in a luxurious mood, but if you prefer to pamper your skin at home, here are three of my favorite methods.

TO DEEP CLEANSE YOUR SKIN

Put 3 tablespoons of oatmeal in a small pouch of muslin, cheesecloth, or gauze. Moisten the oatmeal bag with warm water and rub it all over your face for two minutes. This helps exfoliate the skin and loosen blackheads. Next, apply the wet oatmeal directly to your face, leaving it on for five minutes. This helps to temporarily tighten the skin. Rinse off with warm water. Your face will have a polished glow.

TO WAKE UP YOUR SKIN

After cleansing and towel drying your skin, apply a toner made from equal parts of apple cider vinegar and water. Apply with cotton and let it air dry. This natural toner helps tighten pores temporarily and normalize the skin's pH balance.

TO REJUVENATE YOUR SKIN

Cold plain yogurt applied on clean skin is a superb healing and tightening mask. Leave on for ten to fifteen minutes. Rinse with warm water, then cold. Or, instead of yogurt you can use cold teabags or those old reliable cold, fresh cucumber slices. An ice pack will work, too, and I find it just as soothing as the other remedies.

Eyebrows

Usually, the brow should start directly above the inner corner of the eye. Its highest point should be just beyond the outer edge of the iris, and it should taper to the end. Always tweeze after cleansing and moisturizing the face, then follow with an application of witch hazel or alcohol. I use a pointed-tip tweezer called La Pluck, made by Tweezerman, sold in many beauty supply stores for about twelve dollars. Be sure to sterilize your tweezers with alcohol before using them.

Your eyebrows should *frame* your eyes, not distract from them. Always tweeze from the bottom of the brow, removing all stray hairs. Never pluck brows until they are too thin.

In most cases, I prefer brows to be one or two shades lighter than your hair. If you are very blond or gray, the opposite is true. If your brows need lightening, have them bleached at a salon or try one of the at-home bleaching kits. If you do it yourself, leave the product on for no more than half the time recommended on the package. If your brows are still too dark, do it again. Jolen makes a convenient brow-bleaching kit for under four dollars.

Ready, Set, Glow!

Once your face is clean and moisturized and your brows are tweezed, you're ready to begin your makeup. But if you look in the mirror before you begin, you'll find that your face is beautiful right now. Take a moment to appreciate its special features, the unique tones, the planes and curves that add up to YOU. For now, put aside all criticism; don't worry about the color of your eyes, the length of your nose, or the shape of your face. The perfect face shape is the one you see in the mirror.

Now I'm going to show you first how to flatter that perfectly shaped face with makeup and then, in the next chapter, how to frame it with the right hairdo.

Instant Makeover Magic in Ten Steps

In the rest of this chapter I'll discuss each of the ten steps in the first phase of your instant makeover and I'll show you how each step plays an integral part in the looks of women just like you. Here are the steps we'll cover:

1. Blemish cover
2. Concealer
3. Foundation
4. Highlighter
5. Contour shadow
6. Face powder
7. Blusher
8. Eye makeup
9. Eyebrows
10. Lip color

We'll also cover an optional step, 7A, which involves showing off your nose to its best advantage, but more on that soon enough.

BLEMISH COVER

With your middle finger, gently dot a small amount of neutralizer cream on the areas you wish to conceal.

Covering blemishes, red blotches, sunburned noses, and broken capillaries is easy when you use the right product. Most cosmetic companies offer an off-white cover-up cream or stick that only causes red spots to turn a lighter pink.

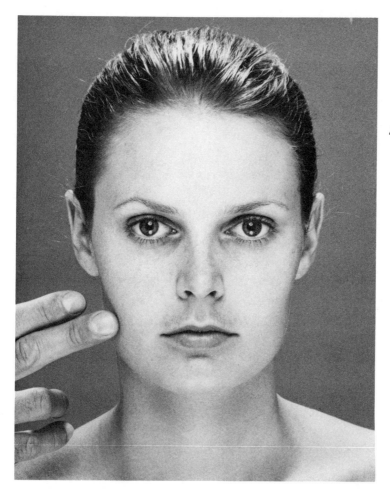

Step 1: Blemish cover

I recommend yellowish cream neutralizer, which covers the red. Ben Nye and William Tuttle, two of the film industry's most famous makeup artists, both offer products that will erase excess redness. Ben Nye's is called Mellow Yellow, and William Tuttle's is Meller Yeller. The products are available at theatrical beauty supply houses, or by writing to Ben Nye (11571 Santa Monica Boulevard, Los Angeles, California 90025) or to William Tuttle (Custom Color Cosmetics, PO Box 56, Pacific Palisades, California 90272).

If you have skin discolorations such as liver spots, scars, or birthmarks, Lydia O'Leary's Covermark, an opaque cream available in various shades, works marvelously to cover them. Originally developed to aid birthmark and burn victims, the product is available in department stores and beauty supply houses. Apply it just as you would a neutralizer, before your foundation.

LYNN REDGRAVE

LYNN'S NATURAL FEATURES
Expressive mouth
Excellent teeth
Bright blue eyes
Good brow line
Strong chin
Nose tends to look wide on camera
Beautiful skin texture
Some blotchiness

Lynn Redgrave's complexion is clear and smooth, with some red blotchiness. Blemish cover camouflages these blotchy areas, creating an even-toned skin surface for her foundation.

With or without makeup, her beautiful blue eyes dance, her smooth skin glows, and her entire image is framed with a sensuous mass of gorgeous red hair.

"I'm five-foot-ten and I love being tall. In fact, when I dress up, I always wear three-inch heels to make myself even taller. My complexion is excellent—no pimples and very small pores—so when I wear makeup, my skin looks beautiful. My lips have a good shape—those are the pluses. But I sometimes suffer from heat splotches, blotchy cheeks, and a red nose—not very glamorous.

"When I really assess my body, I see good legs, but my hips have dips and bumps—cellulite. But I'm not disciplined like Jane Fonda, so I live with my cellulite. I couldn't go through the torture and misery of losing it. The only exercise I get is walking up the hill to my house and climbing the stairs inside."

The mother of three, Lynn is married to her manager, John Clark. Since her pregnancies she has had to keep a keen eye on what she eats, so she follows the Weight Watchers plan. "When I saw *Georgy Girl* on the big screen, I was faced with what other people saw. I looked pretty awful. The camera showed how heavy I was. I wore very little makeup. I decided that only I could improve myself, so I dieted and started wearing makeup. I've come a long way from my sixties look of putting Mary Quant highlights on a baby-fat face."

Although Lynn says she doesn't have any beauty secrets, she admits that she never uses soap on her face. "I use Albolene cream to remove all my makeup, and then moisturize with a cream I buy in England. I rarely go out in the sun, since I don't tan,

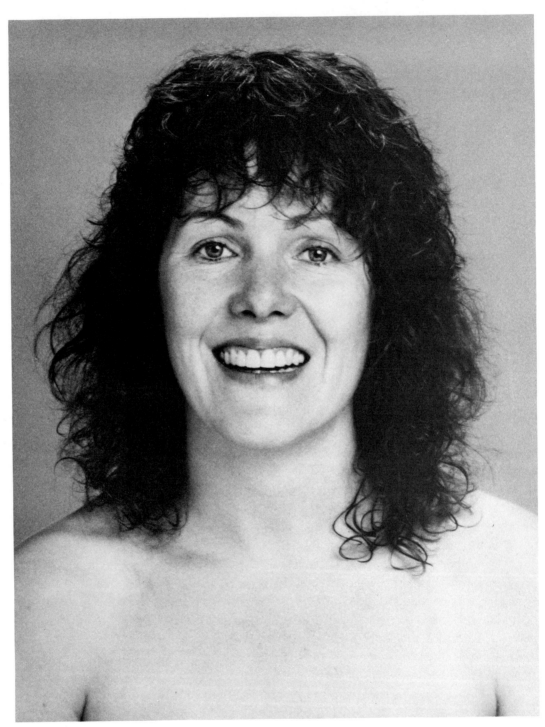

Lynn Redgrave

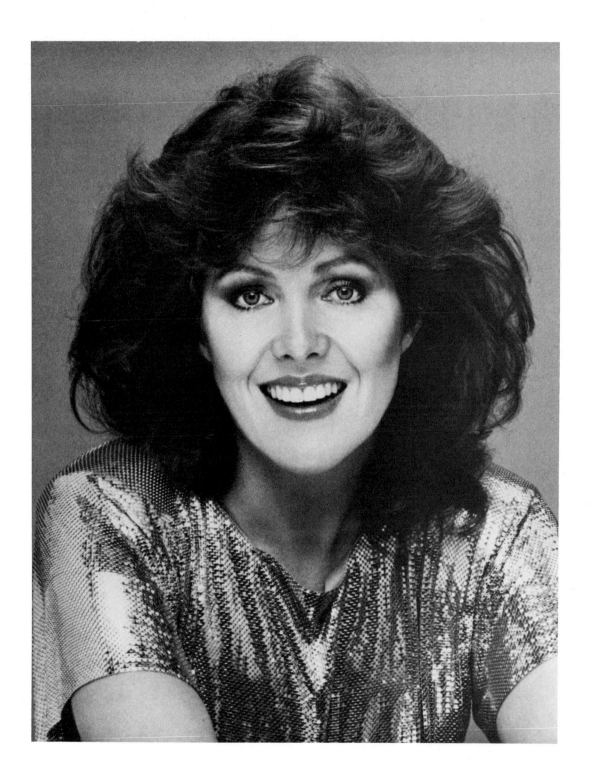

anyway—I just burn. If I *must* be in the sun, I use Sun Dare sun block. I've never had a facial, nor have I ever had a manicure or pedicure, since I hate to wear nail polish. I'm not one to speak to about beauty secrets, am I?"

Lynn's layered haircut, by Jerry Brennen of Vidal Sassoon, adds controlled fullness to her thick, wavy hair. To make the most of Lynn's hair for her photograph, top stylist Hugh York used a blow dryer, a few strategically placed hot rollers, and a round brush. Once he had blow-dried her hair, Hugh used the rollers at the crown and sides to add more bounce. After he removed the rollers, he again used a blow dryer, this time with a round brush, to give Lynn's hair its soft, unstructured look.

Lynn's Makeup

1. Mellow Yellow blemish cover over some of Lynn's reddish areas, especially around her nose and cheeks.
2. No concealer.
3. Light beige liquid foundation.
4. To accent her cheekbones, I blended three dots of liquid highlighter above the cheekbones.
5. Brown contour shadow from in front of the ears to the center of her cheeks below the cheekbones; the same contour shadow on the center of her chin to slightly diminish her prominent chin line.
6. Translucent face powder.
7. Rosy pink blusher on her cheekbones and on the "apples" of her cheeks.
7A. For photography purposes only, shading both sides of her nose and adding a touch of highlighter down the center helps give the nose definition, since a camera takes away some of its dimension. For everyday purposes, Lynn's nose looks terrific and doesn't need contouring. (See optional Step 7A in this chapter.)
8. Plum eye shadow in the crease of her lids extending out and up toward the tip of her brow; light lavender on the lids; darker lavender at the outer corners; muted purple eye liner on the top and bottom lids; black inner liner on the top lids to define the eyes; black eye liner on the outer corners of the eyes, smudged slightly; two coats of black mascara.
9. No brow color.
10. Flesh-tinted highlighter pencil to define the crest of her upper lip; no lip liner; no lipstick, since she has good color in her lips; reddish purple lip gloss.

CONCEALER

With your middle finger, apply a few dots of concealer to the dark areas of your face. Use a flesh-tint eye shadow crayon to lighten any expression lines you want to diminish.

Select a concealer cream (or stick, if you prefer) about two shades lighter than your natural skin tone. Max Factor's Erace is one of the most popular brands, and since it comes in stick form, it's very easy to use.

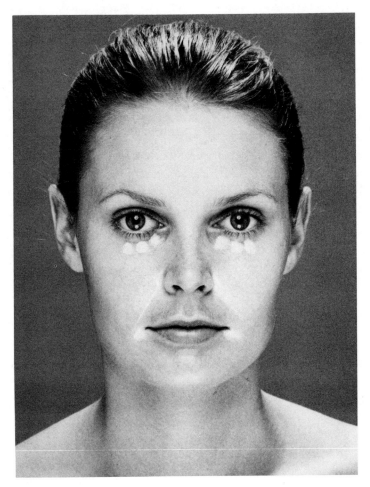

Step 2: Concealer

If you need it, apply the concealer to the bluish gray area directly under the eyes (if you have bags, there's another technique I'll discuss later on), around the outside of the nostrils, below the corners of the mouth, and on the crease of the chin. If the inside corner of the eye and the bridge of the nose seem discolored, concealer can also be used in those spots. Make sure you have applied this light cream to the dark areas only. Blend carefully with your middle finger, patting your under-eye region very lightly.

If your "smile lines" or other expression lines bother you, one very effective trick is to draw right over them. Using a sharpened eye shadow crayon that's a few shades lighter than your skin, or a fine sable brush coated with your concealer cream, color in those lines. Be sure your new light line is as fine as your expression line. Don't blend; applying your foundation will smooth away the lines. Layla, an Italian cosmetics line available at many beauty supply stores, makes an excellent crayon at a very reasonable price.

If you have bags under your eyes, apply a contour shadow cream that's one shade darker than your foundation directly over the bag, and use concealer cream or your light crayon in the crease just under the puffy region.

After you apply foundation (Step 3), you may find that you need to re-apply concealer to further lighten any discolorations. Remember to blend carefully so that this reapplication fades away into your foundation. Concealer should never be too thick, since it can cake after you apply face powder (Step 6).

Concealer can also be used on large freckles or discolorations on the chest and hands. Dot the concealer on the area, blend a bit of foundation over it, and set it with translucent face powder.

CAROL GWENN

CAROL'S NATURAL FEATURES
Skin discoloration
Very round face
Small, deep-set, almond-shaped brown eyes
High cheekbones
Thin brows
Cute, upturned nose
Dimples
Small lips
Thin upper lip
Fleshy chin
A few blemishes

Free-lance writer Carol Gwenn has dark discoloration under her eyes and around her nose. To solve these problems, I used Lydia O'Leary's Covermark, an opaque cream, before applying foundation. She has worn large-size clothing for years and says she has never really found her "look." I showed her how a softer V-neckline, worn with an upturned collar, helps frame her face. Removing the multi-charm necklace allows the eyes to focus on her face; hoop earrings also draw the eyes upward. Carol said her confidence zoomed once she saw how terrific she could look.

Carol's Makeup

1. Blemish cover where necessary.
2. Lydia O'Leary's Covermark over the heavily pigmented areas on the face, especially under the eyes and around the nose.
3. Liquid foundation helps blend the concealer and even out the skin tones.
4. Highlighter above her cheekbones create more angles in her face.
5. Contour shadow applied to the sides of her face to narrow it; darker contour shadow under the cheekbones for definition and under her chin to slim it.
6. Translucent face powder.

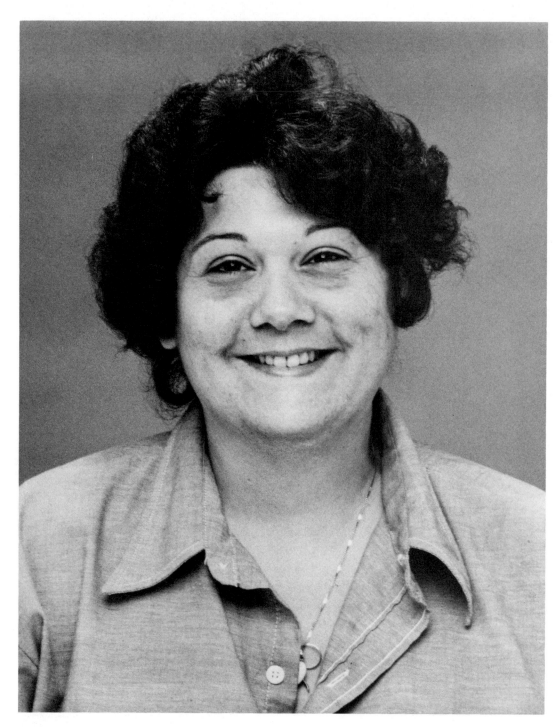

Carol Gwenn

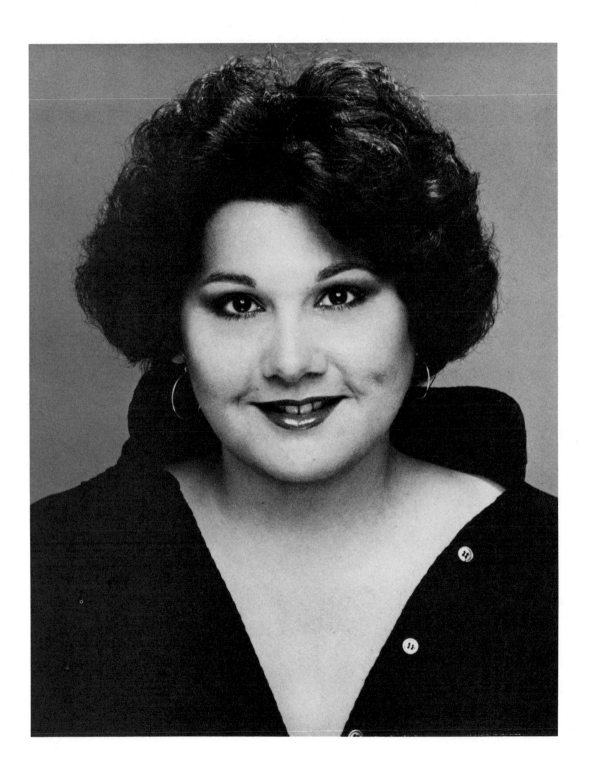

7. Coral blusher on the cheekbones and temples.

7A. Sides of the nose are shaded with neutral brown contour shadow; highlighter is applied in a thin line from the bridge to the tip of the nose.

8. Muted lavender eye shadow at the crease, blended up toward the brow, makes eyes look larger; slate blue eye shadow darkest at the outer corners, slanting upward toward the end of her brow; light pink eye shadow on the center of the eyelid; white inner eye liner on the lower lid to give the illusion of more whites to her eye; black eye liner on the top and bottom lids, smudged slightly; two coats of black mascara.

9. Dark brown and charcoal eyebrow pencils add fullness to her brows.

10. Red lip liner extends slightly outside her natural lip line of her upper lip; red lipstick; gloss.

JANET LEVY

JANET'S NATURAL FEATURES
Discoloration under eyes
Slightly sallow skin tone
Nicely spaced hazel eyes
Dimples
Warm smile

Without makeup, the puffiness under Janet's eyes makes her look older than she is and distracts from her soulful eyes. A few dots of concealer gently blended under each eye covers the discoloration.

Janet is a practicing metaphysician who uses positive thinking to effect changes in her life. "As I feel better and better about myself, that positive attitude shines through me and I start to look better. I've lost weight, changed my gray hair to blond, even got a perm. I've learned not to fear change—never say 'never'—because you *never* know!" Janet's new, lighter hair color complements her skin tones, bringing out a youthful glow that softens her look and brightens her face.

Janet's Makeup

1. No blemish cover was needed.
2. Concealer under eyes and on the smile lines that extend from the edge of the nose to the corners of her mouth.
3. Pinkish beige liquid foundation.
4. No highlighter, because Janet employs a very light, no-makeup look.
5. No contour shadow, for the same reason.
6. Translucent face powder.
7. Peach blusher on the cheekbones.
8. Medium brown eye shadow on the crease of the lid, blended up toward the brow and concentrated in the outer corners; tan shadow on the eyelids; no inner eye liner; dark brown eye liner on the top and very little on the bottom lids, smudged slightly; two coats of dark brown mascara.
9. Light brown eyebrow pencil to fill in the brows and add definition.
10. Light orange-brown lip liner; light orange lipstick; gloss.

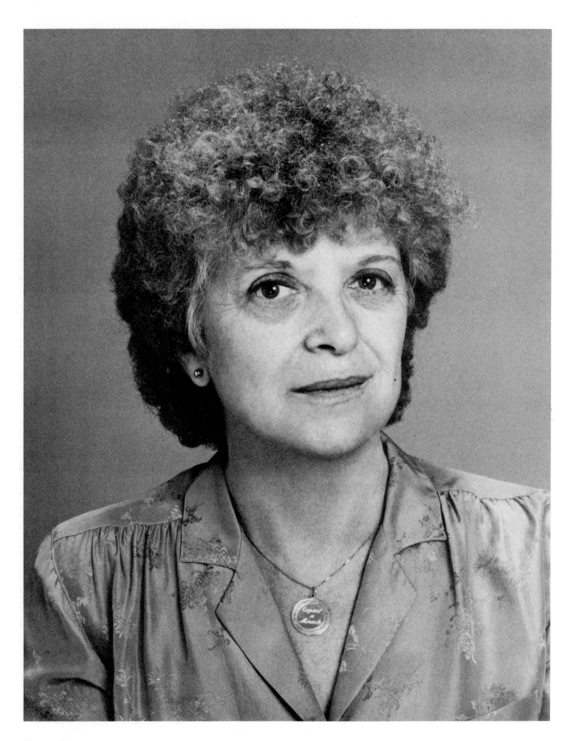

Janet Levy

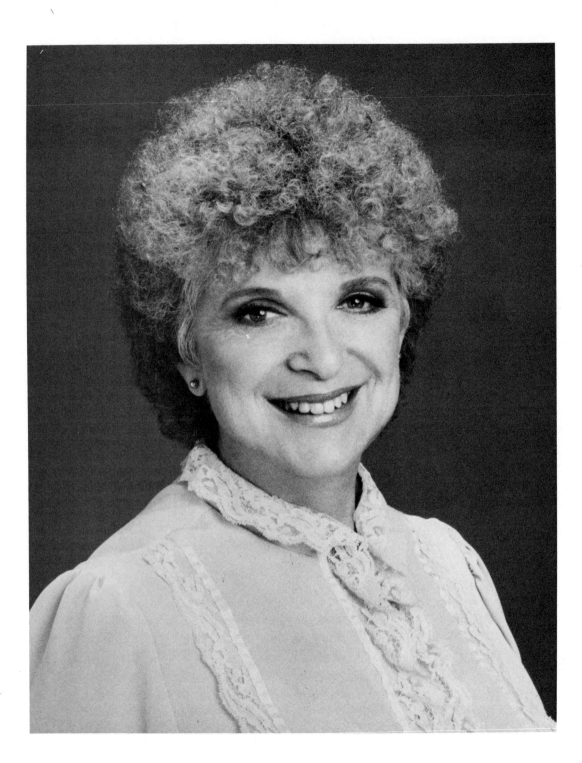

FOUNDATION

Using a latex sponge and liquid foundation, dot your forehead, cheeks, nose, and chin with foundation. Again using your sponge, smooth the dots of makeup out toward your hairline and down toward your neck, covering your entire face ever so lightly with foundation. For even sheerer coverage, dampen your sponge with water first. Don't forget to apply foundation to your eyelids, nostrils, and lips. The coverage should end just below the jawline. Blend carefully to avoid any lines of demarcation.

Most women still have a problem selecting the proper type and shade of foundation for their skin. Use an oil-base liquid foundation if your skin is normal to dry, or a water-base liquid for oily skin. Many cream foundations provide good coverage for skin disclorations.

Don't be afraid to try a number of different types of foundations when you are shopping. Apply them to different parts of your face and see how you like the consistency and coverage. Revlon's Touch & Glow is a comparatively inexpensive oil-base product that is suitable for most slightly dry to normal skin types and offers a nice array of colors. Clinique's Balanced Makeup Base, a water-base product, is excellent for oily or sensitive skin, while Ultima II's CHR Extraordinary Face Makeup, with its special moisturizers, smoothly covers lined and wrinkled skin. For very dry or wrinkled skin, Countess Isserlyn foundation (available at fine department stores) has talc in it and offers a well-covered finish.

I suggest that most women avoid foundations that claim to be iridescent, since these tend to make you look older. If your skin is very wrinkled, avoid all thick cream bases, which can accumulate in the crevices of the wrinkles.

When selecting a foundation, never test the color on your neck or on the back of your hand. Test it where you're going to wear it—on your face. Naturally, you should not be wearing any other foundation at the time. The shade you buy should exactly match your skin tone, unless you are trying to counterbalance your natural sallowness or ruddiness. Women with extremely

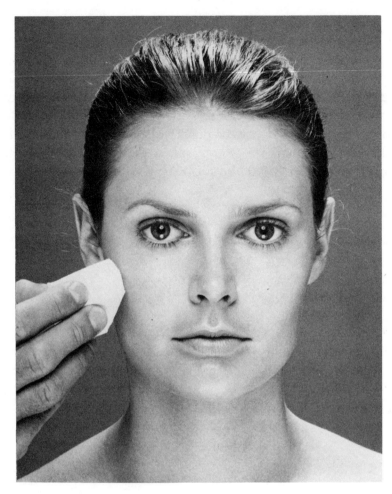

Step 3: Foundation

sallow complexions might prefer a foundation with a hint of pink, while ruddier-skinned types may opt for a foundation with a slightly yellow cast. This can be tricky, so when in doubt, go for the shade that exactly matches your skin and then simply use a blusher to counterbalance your skin tone. (More about blushers later.)

I suggest that black women avoid a rosy foundation, since many have blue or ashen undertones in their complexion, and a rosy foundation looks unnatural. Barbara Walden's line of cosmetics for black women offers a variety of shades, many of which have orange undertones that are more complimentary.

There are dozens of brands of foundation available in most drug stores and department stores, as well as many private-label products made by skin specialists who have their own companies. But are you aware that there are several brands of theatrical makeup that are often exactly the same as those made by cosmetics companies but much less expensive? I've mentioned Ben Nye's products and William Tuttle's line, Custom Color Cosmetics, but there are many others available at beauty supply stores and theatrical beauty supply centers and by mail. A brochure about various theatrical makeup products and a list of places where they may be purchased can be obtained by writing to Doris Butler at Columbia Drug Store, one of the largest sources of theatrical makeup in Hollywood (1440 North Gower, California 90028).

MARIETTE HARTLEY

MARIETTE'S NATURAL FEATURES
Low brow bone
Freckles
Deep-set blue eyes
Reddish undertones to her skin
Dimples
Narrow nose
Defined, high cheekbones

If your freckles are part of your personality, why hide them? Use a sheer foundation like I've used on Mariette Hartley, and let your freckles glow. This will help to even the skin tones without covering up something so intrinsically charming.

Study Mariette's before photo and note the features that cosmetics will define: high cheekbones, a well-shaped nose, and bright eyes. A touch of makeup enhances all of them without taking away her natural freshness.

"I like my freckles to show—I'd really lose a part of me if I didn't have my freckles," says Mariette. "I've never had a hangup about freckles, even as a child. My hangup was that I hated my legs. My dad used to tease me about them. In fact, he taught me how to whistle because he told me that with my legs I'd never be able to get a cab in New York. As I grew up, they became much more shapely—now I even have ankles!"

When Mariette first started at MGM in the early 1960s, the typical female star's image was that of a voluptuous creature who wore lots of makeup and exuded glamour. Uncomfortable with that role but eager to pursue her career, Mariette was relieved when the natural look became the vogue. As soon as she began doing commercials, she mastered her own makeup and hair and found that enhancing her *own* look worked the best.

As part of her regular skin preservation routine, Mariette gets facials at least twice a month, a program she began shortly after the birth of her first child. At that time, her skin seemed to lose its glow and needed the deep cleaning and stimulation of frequent facials. Now she considers her trips to the skin care salon a luxurious way to relax. "If I had more time, I'd have a facial once a week," says the statuesque, five-foot-eight-and-three-quarter-inch blonde. At home she uses Prescription Plus cosmetics and chooses a liquid cleanser instead of soap for her face. Once or twice a week she uses a granular scrub to slough off old, dry skin cells. She always wears her hair in a soft, natural style, much

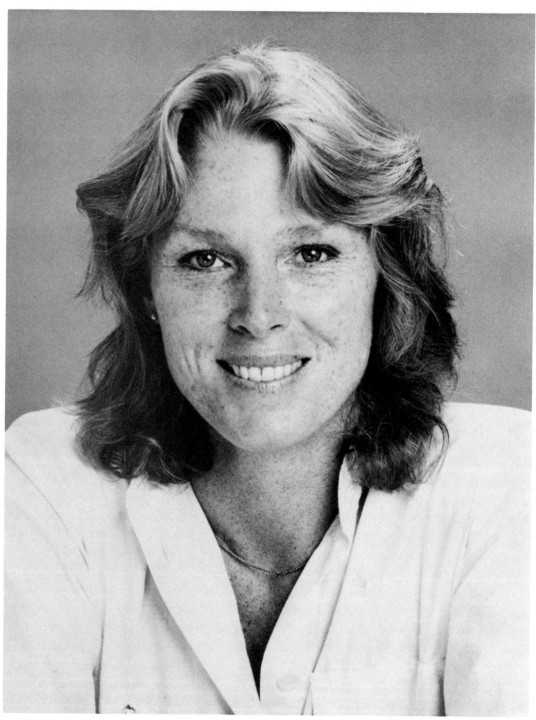

Mariette Hartley

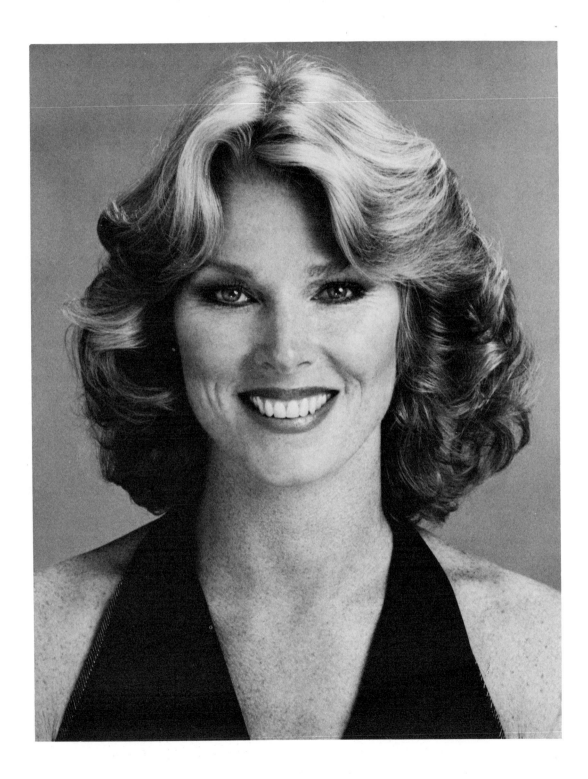

like the one Studio City stylist Barron created for her after photo. With just a few hot rollers and a little back brushing, her otherwise limp hair appears fuller.

"Sure, I'd like to have larger breasts, thinner legs, smaller feet, beautiful hands, and long, long hair that didn't fall out with every pregnancy, but I've learned to like just being myself."

Mariette's Makeup

1. No blemish cover.
2. No concealer.
3. Beige liquid foundation with a slight yellow cast to balance the red tones in her skin.
4. A touch of highlighter above her cheekbones.
5. No contour shadow.
6. Translucent face powder.
7. Rosy pink blusher on her cheekbones, on her chin, and across the bridge of her nose.
8. Purple eye shadow in the crease of the lid; light lavender shadow on the entire lid, blending the color up toward her brow, deemphasizing her low brow bone; extra shadow at the outside corners of the eyes; no inner eye liner; charcoal liner on the upper and lower lids, smudged slightly; two coats of black mascara.
9. Light brown and silverized beige brow pencils in feathery strokes, then blended.
10. Light brown lip liner; neutral beige lipstick; gloss.

SANDRA MARSHALL

SANDRA'S NATURAL FEATURES
Smooth, freckled complexion
High forehead
High cheekbones
Very light lashes and brows
Ample space between eyes and brows
Expressive, large, steel blue eyes
Nose fleshy toward tip
Nicely shaped lips, large mouth
Square jawline
Small chin

Actress Sandra Marshall has one of those faces that changes with the slightest application of makeup. Everything about her is pale, so the least bit of color makes a big difference. Though I often recommend that women with freckles let them show, Sandra's were too light to show up as more than tiny blotches on her otherwise beautiful complexion. A cream foundation provides enough coverage to even out the tones of her skin and create a wonderful porcelain finish.

Sandra's Makeup

1. No blemish cover.
2. Some concealer under eyes and at lines from nostrils to outside corners of the mouth.
3. Beige cream foundation to eliminate freckles.
4. Highlighter to accent her already prominent cheekbones and bring her chin forward; highlighter at inner corner of the eyes.
5. Contour shadow under her cheekbones to emphasize them; contour shadow on the temples to slim her face slightly.
6. Translucent face powder.
7. Peach blusher on her cheekbones and temples and across the bridge of her nose.

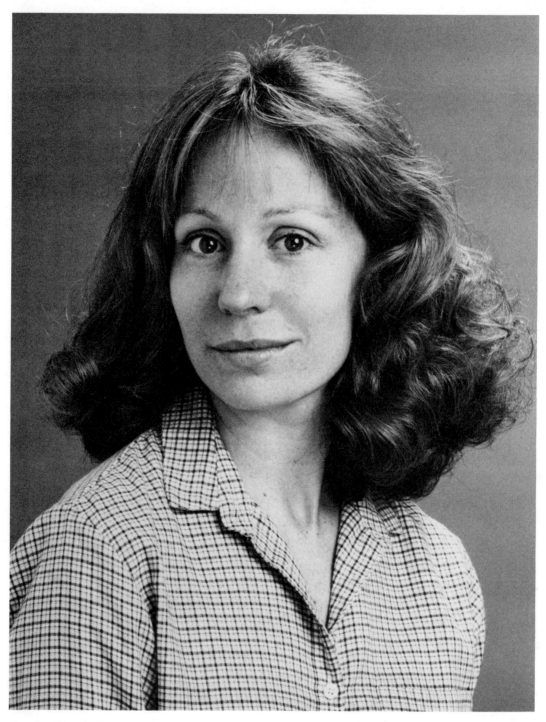

Sandra Marshall

7A. The sides of her nose are shaded with neutral brown contour shadow powder; highlighter powder is applied in a thin line from the bridge of the nose to the tip; all are carefully blended.

8. Sandy brown eye shadow darkens the crease of her eyelid and extends out and up toward the tip of the brow; gray eye shadow is concentrated in the outer corners of her eyes; light beige shadow in the inner corners to create the illusion of wider-set eyes; light blue inner eye liner on the lower inner lid only to bring out the blue in her eyes; charcoal eye liner on the upper and lower lids, smudged slightly; two coats of black mascara.

9. Silverized beige and light brown eyebrow pencils to create a higher arch to her brows and slightly extend their length.

10. Medium brown lip liner; dark beige lipstick; gloss.

JUNE ALLYSON

JUNE'S NATURAL FEATURES
Narrow, deep-set dark blue eyes
Light lashes
Tiny nose
Warm smile, good teeth
Fine, thin hair

June Allyson doesn't wear foundation when she isn't working. Since her skin is slightly dry with uneven skin tones, a foundation evens it and gives her a dewy glow. It's a simple but noticeable change.

When I think of June Allyson, I automatically smile. Clichéd as it may sound, to know her is to love her. The petite star (she's just a hair over five feet and weighs only ninety-eight pounds) started her career at MGM when she was fifteen, and it wasn't long before she was Mrs. Dick Powell. The pair became a Hollywood legend. When he died, she felt that her world was shattered. "I was a widow at an early age, and I was lost. I felt there was no world left for me." Eventually, she says, "I learned how to stop feeling sorry for myself and to *take care* of myself. Now I'm very happy."

June's wearing her hair the same way she wore it when she was one year old—and she has pictures to prove it! To add fullness, stylist Hugh York used a medium-diameter round hairbrush and a blow dryer, curling the sides toward her face.

June recalls her early days at MGM: "When I first started, they told me that I was just what they were looking for but that I had a lisp, a very strange voice, and that my smile made my eyes disappear. So they sent me to specialists to correct everything. The voice coach expelled me, the dentist refused to touch my beautiful, healthy teeth, and the eye specialist said, 'That's just what happens when you smile.' So now, when I meet young actors and actresses—or anyone, for that matter—I tell them to pick out their best features, enhance them and don't try to get rid of the things that make you different from everyone else."

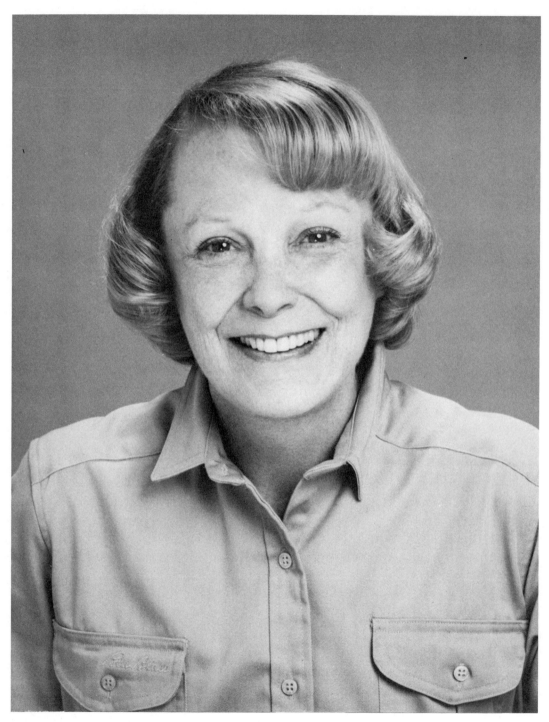

June Allyson

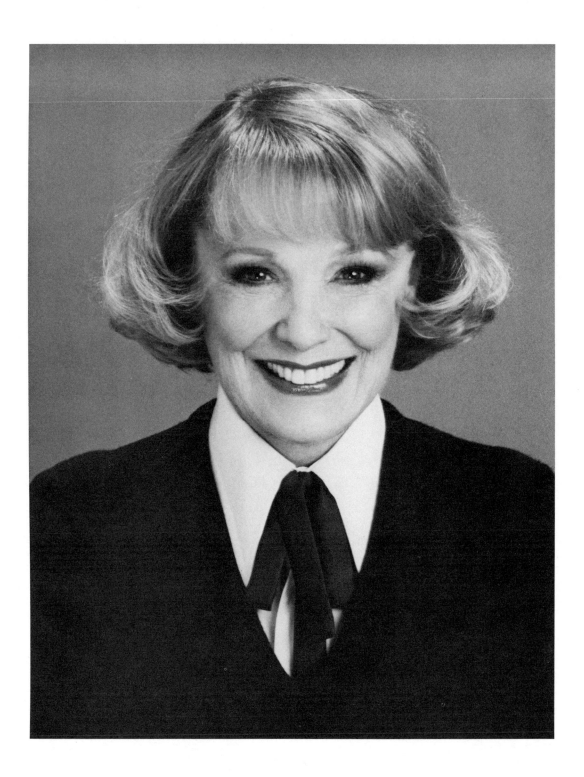

1. No blemish cover.
2. Concealer in the inner corners of the eyes and under the eyes.
3. Rosy beige liquid foundation.
4. Highlighter above the cheekbones and on the eyelids to bring out her deep-set eyes.
5. Very little contour shadow under her cheekbones.
6. Translucent face powder.
7. Peach blusher on the "apples" of her cheeks.
8. Brown eye shadow in the crease of the lid and above it to create a rounder illusion for the eye; slate blue shadow on the outer corners of the lid; no inner eye liner; charcoal eye liner on the top and bottom lids, smudged slightly; a strip of artificial lashes on the top lid only; one coat of black mascara.
9. Silverized beige eyebrow pencil.
10. Orange-beige lip liner; light orange-brown lipstick; gloss.

HIGHLIGHTER

With your fingertips, apply three dots of highlighter cream above each cheekbone. To blend, pat—don't rub—with your middle finger, extending the highlighter toward the temple.

Since highlighter reflects light, it will make your cheekbones appear more prominent. If your chin recedes, highlighter will help to bring it forward. Be aware, however, that highlighter used too low on the cheeks will make them

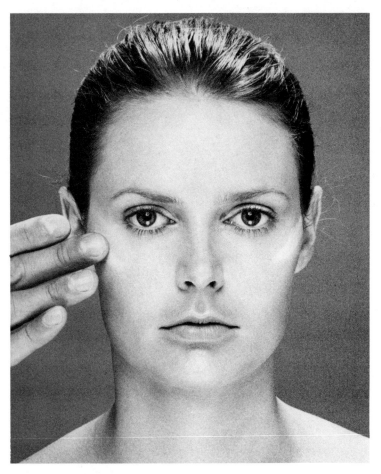

Step 4: Highlighter

look pudgy, and highlighter dabbed on a strong chin will make it appear too prominent. Sparingly applied, highlighter can do wonders for your face.

Select a highlighter that is about two shades lighter than your skin tone. It should never be pure white, since white makeup often takes on a bluish cast. A foundation two or three shades lighter than your skin works very well as a highlighter.

Although I prefer cream highlighter, there are powder versions that work well. Lancôme's Dual Finish Creme/Powder Makeup is excellent. If you choose a powder highlighter, use it after you've applied your translucent face powder (Step 6), and always apply with a sable brush. For dramatic evenings, you might like the effect of an iridescent powder or gel used on your cheekbones, on the brow bone, or just above your brows.

MARILU HENNER

MARILU'S NATURAL FEATURES
Full brows
Small, light blue eyes
Slightly wide nose
Flawless complexion
Thin upper lip
Wide jawbone

Marilu Henner, who played Elaine Nardo on "Taxi," has a well-defined face but needed to balance her strong jawbone. Highlighter above the cheekbones and on the tip of her chin made these areas look more prominent. A bit of highlighter applied between the inner corner of her eyes and the bridge of her nose created the illusion of wider-set eyes. Stylist Eric Root blow-dried Marilu's wavy hair using a large, round brush.

Marilu is a devout vegetarian. Her idea of "pigging out" is a rice cake with honey on it. She exercises three times a week using the Pilates method, an exercise technique that combines body balancing and strict concentration. Her intense program includes long and short walks, rigorous aerobics classes, and two hours a day of weight training. She can actually do about 1,000 sit-ups on an incline bench—that means with her head lower than her feet. Her body is an admirable reflection of her discipline.

After struggling for years with acne, Marilu won the battle with good skin care. She uses Aubrey Organics skin cleanser from a neighborhood health food store, follows with an oatmeal scrub, and uses Beverly Hills skin care specialist Nance Mitchell's moisturizer. Marilu sees Nance regularly for facials.

Her best beauty secret? Every day before applying her makeup, Marilu rubs her face with an ice cube.

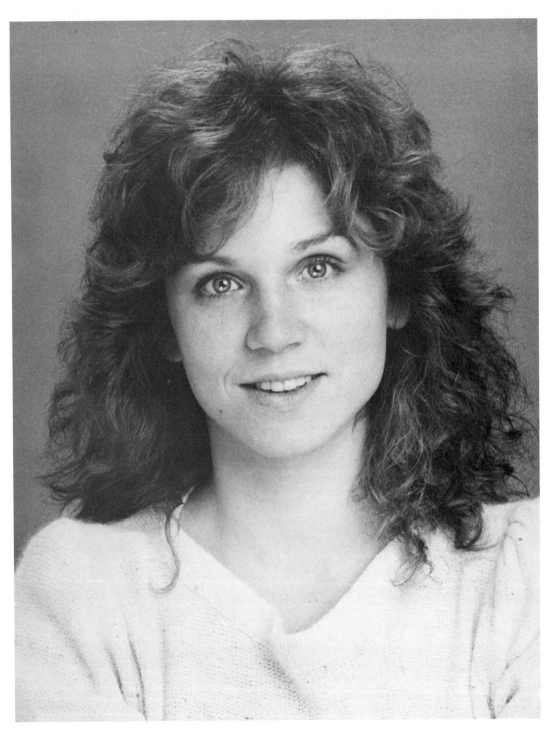

Marilu Henner

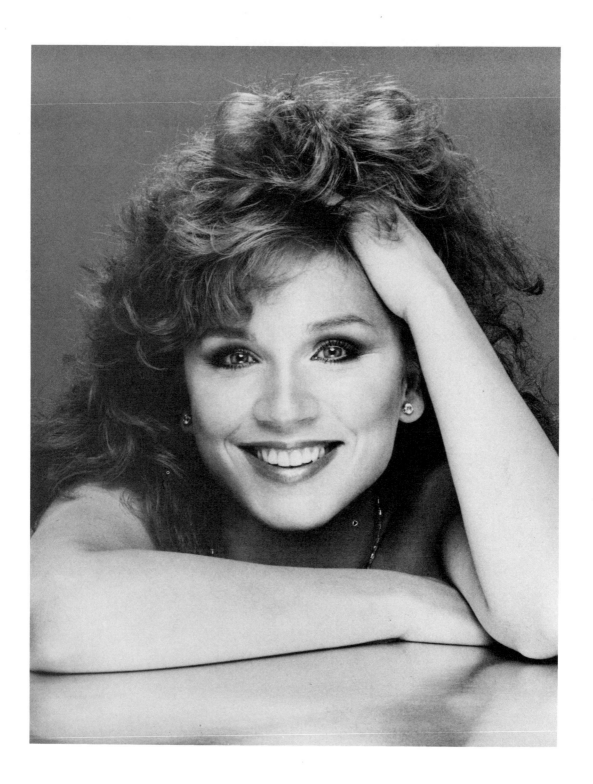

1. No blemish cover.
2. No concealer.
3. Light beige liquid foundation.
4. Highlighter above cheekbones and on center of chin.
5. Contour shadow under cheekbones, blended down to jawline to diminish her prominent jawbone.
6. Translucent face powder.
7. Pink blusher on cheekbones.
7A. Sides of the nose shaded with neutral brown contour shadow powder; highlighter powder applied in a thin line from the bridge of the nose to the tip; all carefully blended.
8. Muted purple eye shadow in the crease of the lid; light lavender shadow on the lid; no shadow on the brow bone; light blue inner eye liner on bottom to make eyes look larger and bluer; black eye liner on top and on bottom outer corners, smudged; two coats of black mascara.
9. Light brown eyebrow pencil to fill in her brows.
10. Reddish purple lip liner extending outside her natural lip line on both upper and lower lips to make her mouth appear fuller; reddish purple lipstick; lip gloss.

ERIN GRAY

ERIN'S NATURAL FEATURES
Beautiful blue eyes
Eyes can appear close set
Face can appear narrow
Straight nose, nice profile
High cheekbones
Slightly thin upper lip
Perfect teeth

When Erin Gray and I first met, she mentioned that her face lacked a strong bone structure—she felt she needed lots of makeup. I told her that more highlighter would solve the problem. She has a narrow face, so I used highlighter on her jawline and immediately below the hollow of her cheeks to help widen the look of her face.

Erin, who co-starred on the "Buck Rogers" TV series and was a sought-after cover girl before landing her role on the comedy series "Silver Spoons," says she spent years practicing how to perfect her look. "People think that models just have pretty faces, put on makeup, and look gorgeous. But that's crazy. We get beauty tips from every makeup artist we meet. We practice on each other. We're overly critical of our faces. But we have to be."

When she's not working, Erin wears little makeup—some blusher, a light shade of gloss, mascara, and occasionally a touch of brown eye shadow. "I've learned to change my makeup depending on where I am. If I'm in New York, I wear a lot more makeup, because the city itself has a gray tinge to it and I need more color. In California, where the sun is bright, I wear brighter color but less of it. I also find that in California I have to take better care of my skin. The sun is so drying. I use La Prairie moisturizer and try to avoid being out in the sun as much as possible. To clean my skin, I use Ivory or Neutrogena soap, rinse with hot water, and follow with a splash of icy cold water."

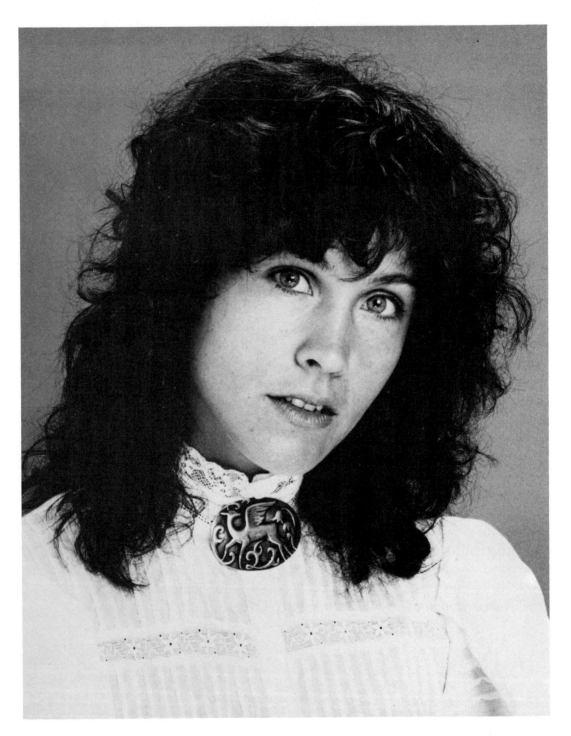

Erin Gray

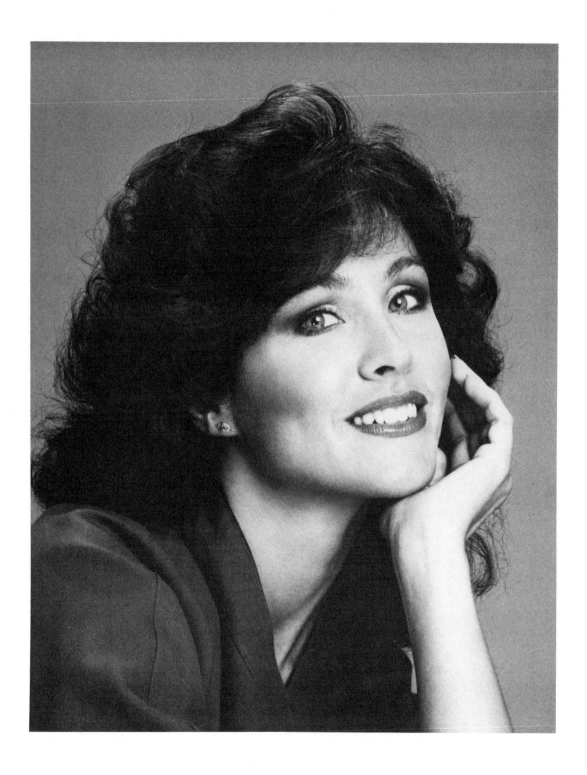

1. No blemish cover.
2. No concealer.
3. Beige liquid foundation.
4. Highlighter above the cheekbones to make her face appear broader, on the eyelids—from the inner corner of the eye to the center of the lid—to make the eyes appear wider set, and below the contour shadow to add more width to her face.
5. Contour shadow below the cheekbones.
6. Translucent face powder.
7. Coral blusher on the "apple" of her cheeks.
8. Medium brown eye shadow in the crease of the lid and intensified at the outer corners to make the eyes appear to be wider set; light peach shadow on the lid and on the brow bone; no inner eye liner; charcoal eye liner at the outer corners of the top and bottom lids, smudged slightly; two coats of black mascara.
9. No eyebrow pencil.
10. Reddish brown lip liner extending slightly outside the natural line of the upper lip; reddish brown lipstick; gloss.

MERRYL JAYE

MERRYL'S NATURAL FEATURES
Small face
Very hollow cheeks
High cheekbones
Small, close-set, deep-set hazel eyes
Porcelain white complexion
Naturally curly red hair
Full lips

Singer/songwriter Merryl Jaye has very hollow cheeks. Although it's unconventional, I applied highlighter to the hollows of her cheeks, where ordinarily contour shadow (Step 5) is applied. This helps create the illusion of a fuller face.

Merryl used to spend dozens of hours of her adult life straightening her curly auburn hair. One day she realized how beautiful those natural curls could be and let her hair grow out in all its glory. In fact, in a few months, her beautiful, tiny face was lost in a mass of fluffy red hair. Pinning it back and allowing some of the tendrils to fall frontward creates a soft romantic look that emphasizes her marvelous cheekbones.

Merryl's Makeup

1. No blemish cover.
2. Concealer under the eyes.
3. Very light liquid foundation.
4. Highlighter used inside the hollows of her cheeks to slightly diminish her sunken look.
5. No contour shadow.
6. Translucent face powder.
7. Soft peach blusher on her cheekbones and chin.
8. Muted green eye shadow extended beyond the outside corners of her eyes to make them appear longer. Darker green eye shadow was applied to the outer corners of her eyes to make them appear farther apart; highlighter on her lids and at the inner corner near the nose to bring out her deep-set

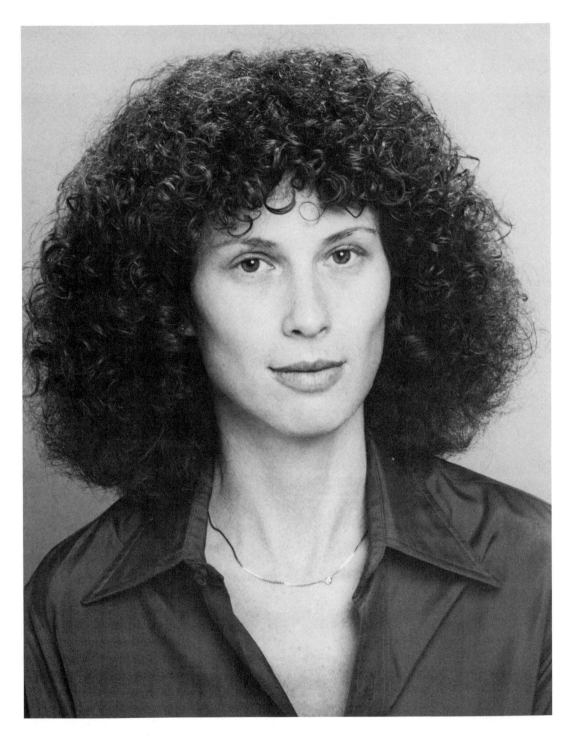

Merryl Jaye

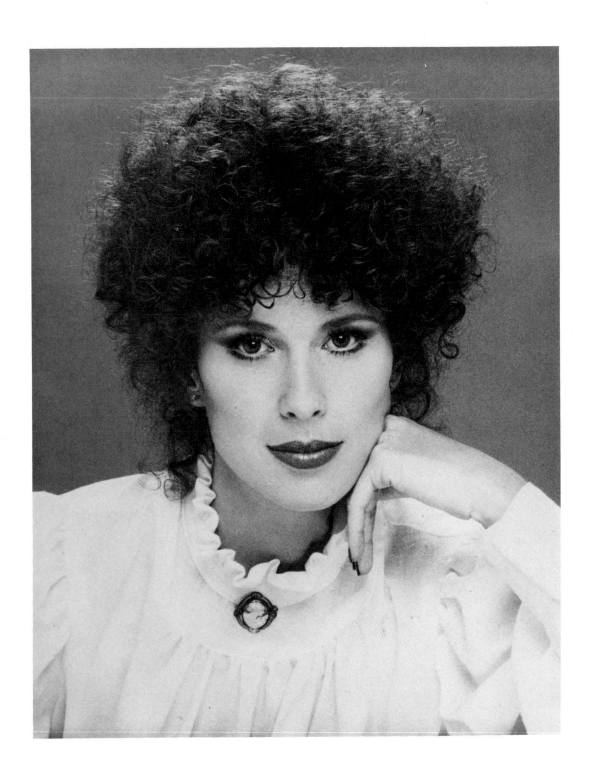

eyes; muted green eye liner, smudged; white lower inner eye liner to create the illusion of having more white area to her eye; two coats of dark brown mascara.

9. Auburn and light brown eyebrow pencils.
10. Orange-brown lipstick; gloss.

CONTOUR SHADOW

Suck in your cheeks and apply a thin band of contour shadow cream in the hollow under your cheekbones and place a small dot on each temple. With your middle finger, blend the contour shadow cream diagonally outward toward the ears. Keep blending until you see a subtle shadow.

Now that you have created some beautiful planes in your face by adding highlighter, it's time to continue the process of sculpting by complementing these light areas with shadow. But before we proceed, I want to caution you. Contour shadow can produce wonderful, dramatic effects in photographs. It can add beautiful subtle shading at night. By day it can make your face look too angular and overly made up, unless you are very meticulous in the blending process. I prefer that women not use contour shadow in the daytime, because I see too few who know how to use it. If you blend carefully, keeping in mind that less is more, you can wear it by day and still effect a subtle look— but be careful.

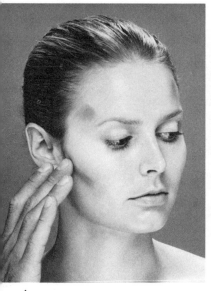 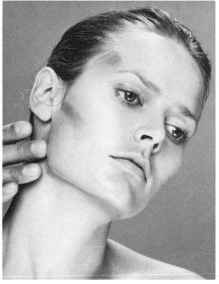 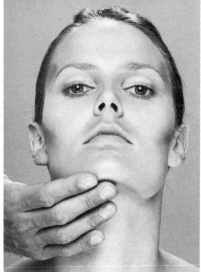

A   B   C

Step 5: Contour shadow

Always remember that any light area appears to come forward, while dark areas seem to recede. A contour shadow should be a very neutral color, a cross between brown and gray, with no red or yellow undertones. Select a contour shadow color that is about two shades darker than your foundation. (Ben Nye makes a color called Subtle Brown which is perfect for most fair skin.) Any darker and you'll look as if you have a dirty face rather than one that's nicely contoured. If you prefer, you may use a liquid foundation in place of a contour shadow cream. Again, I prefer cream because it allows for better control. There are also pressed powder contour shadows, which I recommend for contouring the nose, a trick I save until later (see optional Step 7A). If you choose to use a powder, be sure to use a soft sable brush to apply it.

Blending is very important when using contour shadow. If you have a question about whether you're wearing too much contour shadow, you probably are. Blend again (I like to use my free hand as a blotter to remove excess cream from my finger as I apply). Blend the contour shadow under the cheekbone diagonally outward toward the ear. Be careful not to blend the shadow up into the highlight cream. If your cheekbones are naturally prominent or if your cheeks are already pleasantly hollow, contour shadow is usually unnecessary.

I repeat, unless you are very skilled at applying it, contour shadow should be reserved for evening. The only way to become skilled at contouring is to practice. Start with as little contour shadow as possible—you can always add more. Once you master its application, you can experiment shading other areas.

- To define the jawline, apply contour shadow cream along the underside of the jawbone and blend (see photo B).
- To diminish a double chin, use a dark contour shadow directly under the center of the chin and blend down toward the throat (see photo C).
- To slim a very round face, shade the sides of the face, blending from under the cheekbone downward toward the jawline.
- To soften a square face or a face with a very prominent jawbone, simply shade the sides of the face along the jawbone area, blending downward.

JULIET PROWSE

JULIET'S NATURAL FEATURES
Round face
High forehead
Heavy lids
Large, wide-set, almond-shaped brown eyes
Slightly flat nose
Light lashes and brows
Full lips

Juliet has a round face that can appear too plump without contour shadow—especially when she's in front of the camera. To slim her face, I used contour shadow on the sides of her face and on her temples. To create the illusion of hollow cheeks, I applied the shadow under her cheekbones and blended back toward her ears.

Born in Bombay, India, and raised in Johannesburg, South Africa, Juliet has been dancing since she was six years old. Her fabulous legs and gorgeous body are proof that it pays to work out.

Juliet's fortunate; exercise is second nature to her. She dances every day, without fail. "As a professional dancer, I'm always concerned about my physical appearance. Fortunately, I have the discipline, out of necessity, to keep physically active every day. I find that moving to keep my body tight has other positive effects on me: The constant sweating keeps my skin clear and stimulated, and I have a great deal of energy. I appear much taller than I am—five-feet-seven inches—because of my posture. My mother, who still has perfect posture at seventy-two, taught me at an early age to keep my body in alignment, and my dancing has reinforced it. Naturally, my muscle tone is good—I can always tell a dancer by his or her muscle tone."

In addition to several hours of dancing every day, Juliet attends regular yoga classes with yogi Bikram Choudury. "The classes are far more intense than any dance class I've ever taken," Juliet explains. "Yoga is an excellent mental discipline as well as a physical one and teaches me to have control over every muscle in my body.

"I never wear makeup when I'm working out," Juliet says. "I want my skin to be clean and free of anything that might clog my pores. I use regular soap and Vaseline Intensive Care Lotion as an all-over moisturizer—for my face as well as my body. Occasionally, I apply vitamin E oil. When my skin needs deep cleaning, I get vacuum facials at the Face Place in Los Angeles."

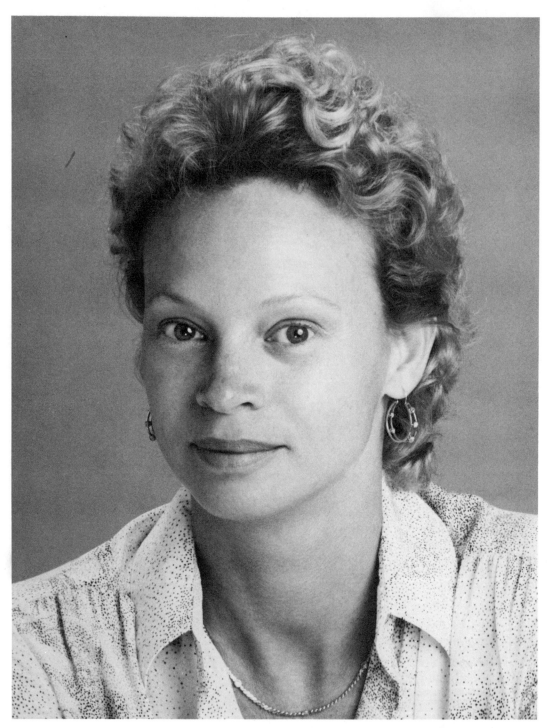

Juliet Prowse

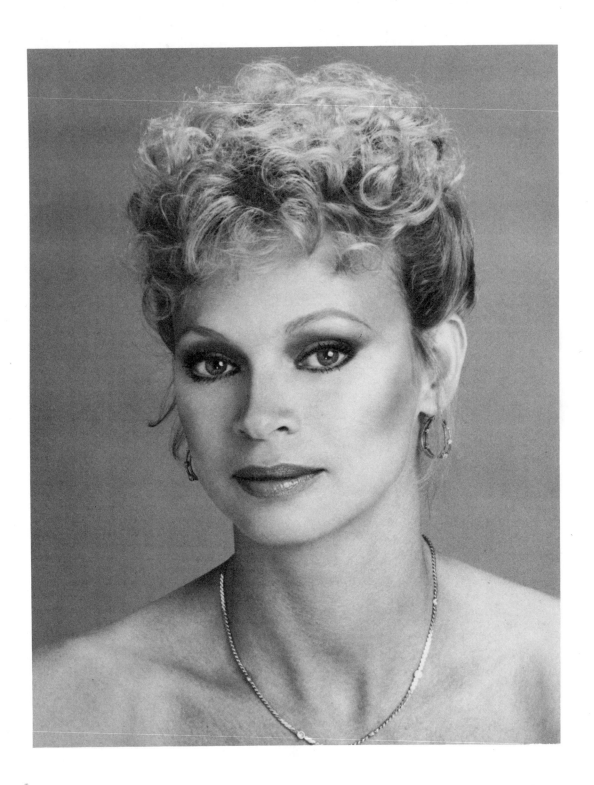

Juliet has fine hair, so super-stylist Ramsey piled her curls on top of her head to make it look thicker and also to add extra length to her round face. "Because of the intense perspiration, I always wear wigs when I work on stage. My natural hair color is a dirty blond with red highlights, but I've kept it red since I was fourteen—my mother suggested the change."

To relax, Juliet gardens, does needlepoint, and reads extensively. She takes great pride in her gourmet cooking skills. "I love salads and stay away from desserts, since I have a tendency to gain weight (that's another reason I keep dancing)," she says.

Asked if there is anything she'd like to change about herself, Juliet laughed and nodded. "I wish I could be more patient, and I'd like to have boobs—I always wanted to have a pair of boobs. But as a dancer, they'd only get in the way, wouldn't they?"

Juliet's Makeup

1. No blemish cover.
2. No concealer.
3. No foundation.
4. Highlighter above the cheekbones to create the illusion of angles.
5. To slim her face, contour shadow below her cheekbones, on the sides of her face, and on the temples.
6. Translucent face powder.
7. Peach blusher.
7A. Sides of the nose shaded with neutral brown contour shadow; highlighter is applied in a thin line from the bridge of the nose to the tip; all carefully blended.
8. Golden tan eye shadow in the crease of the lid; darker golden tan shadow on the lid to minimize the heavy lid; lighter golden tan shadow above the crease, blending it up toward the brow bone; shimmery gold shadow on the brow bone; black inner eye liner at top; black eye liner on top and bottom lids; two coats of black mascara.
9. Silverized beige and light brown eyebrow pencils, blended lightly, to add a touch of color.
10. Orange-brown lip liner; orange-brown lipstick, gold lipstick on the center of lower lip; gloss.

JAYNE KENNEDY

JAYNE'S NATURAL FEATURES
Flawless, even skin
High forehead
Thick brows
Large, catlike brown eyes
High cheekbones
Straight nose
Long chin

When you look at Jayne's before photo, it's difficult to imagine her looking prettier, isn't it? But she's the first to mention her chin, which she feels is too long. With contour shadow on the tip, blended carefully, her chin immediately looks proportionate to the rest of her extraordinary face.

A busy actress and frequent guest on TV talk shows, this five-foot-ten-inch beauty says she wishes she could do something about her height. "It's hard to find clothes that fit properly, and until very recently, it was impossible to find pretty, flat shoes. I wish I were about two inches shorter."

Jayne practices yoga and does aerobic exercise to keep her body in good physical condition. She says her exercise record, *Love Your Body,* is one of her favorite projects. Jane diets carefully. She stays away from fried foods, which, she says, tend to cause her to gain weight and make her skin too oily.

To counteract occasional oiliness, Jayne uses Ivory soap and water on her face. She uses Fashion Fair cosmetics, Oil of Olay as a moisturizer, and Jergens lotion all over her body, including her face.

Jayne conditions her naturally thick hair once a month. When it feels especially dry, she washes it just before bed, applies a protein-rich conditioner, wraps her head in a towel, and goes to sleep. Then she shampoos with a pH-balanced product in the morning. Michelle Lavee blow dried her hair for that straight-hair look. Jayne uses no chemical treatments on her hair.

Does she think she's beautiful? "I never think of myself in those terms. But I love it when young kids come up to me and say that they'd like to grow up to be like me. For me, one of the biggest compliments is to have someone think I'm a nice person—that's when they're really saying I'm beautiful."

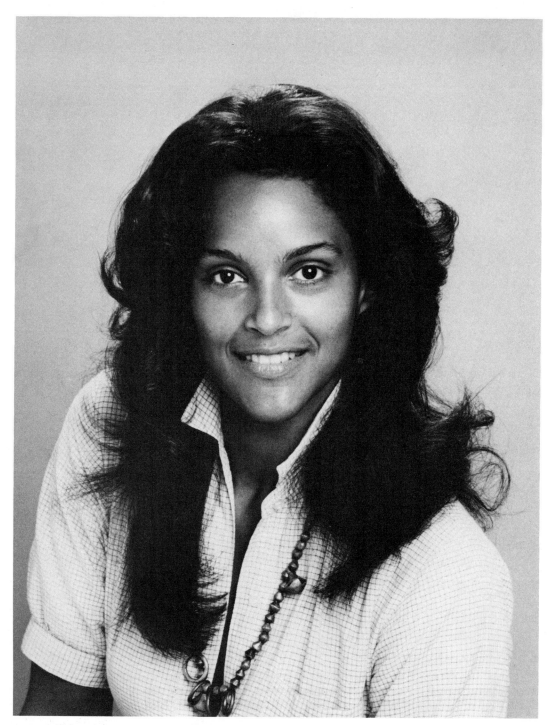

Jayne Kennedy

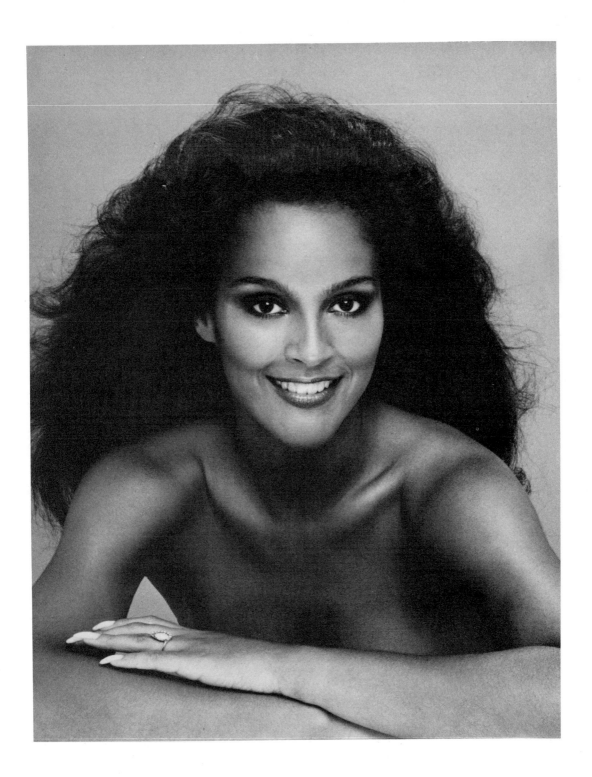

1. No blemish cover.
2. Concealer under the eyes.
3. Dark tan liquid foundation.
4. Highlighter above the cheekbones, blended upward into the temple area to make her eyes look more slanted.
5. Contour shadow in the hollow of her cheeks and on the tip of her chin to minimize its length.
6. Translucent face powder.
7. Earthy red blusher on her cheeks and temples and also across the bridge of her nose and on her chin.
8. Dark brown eye shadow in the crease of the lid, applied outward and upward, intensified at outer corners; golden brown shadow on the lid; just a touch of golden brown shadow on the brow bone; black inner eye liner top and bottom; black eye liner top and bottom; three coats of black mascara.
9. No eyebrow pencil; eyebrows brushed up.
10. Reddish brown lip liner; reddish brown lipstick; gloss.

VICTORIA HEARST

VICTORIA'S NATURAL FEATURES
Beautiful, pale complexion
Dark eyebrows
Wide-set, large brown eyes
Full cheeks
Slightly receding, fleshy chin
Thin lips

Victoria Hearst is an athletic woman with a trim build. However, she has a full face and a fleshy chin that tend to make her look more plump than she is. Contour shadow along her jawline, blended carefully until it almost fades away, diminishes the fleshy look. To define her cheekbones, I used contour shadow on her full cheeks. She hasn't lost the youthful look of her face, but the subtle shadowing has given her a more sophisticated image.

Victoria has a black belt in karate, teaches martial arts, and loves horseback riding and dressing up for glamorous evenings. "I love to look totally feminine by night, but when I work I need a fresh natural look," explains the granddaughter of the late publishing mogul William Randolph Hearst. Victoria has an active social life outside her work and asked for a sophisticated look that would take her easily from dinner to theater to party.

Victoria's long straight hair needs a lift from hot rollers for body. Russell Elliott set her hair in large rollers, back brushed the crown and swept it all off to one side for a glamorous, evening look.

Victoria's Makeup

1. Blemish cover where necessary.
2. No concealer.
3. Water-base liquid foundation for her oily skin.
4. Highlighter above her cheekbones to create definition and highlighter on her chin to help produce a stronger, more pronounced effect.
5. Contour shadow under her cheekbones; also under her chin and along the jawline.

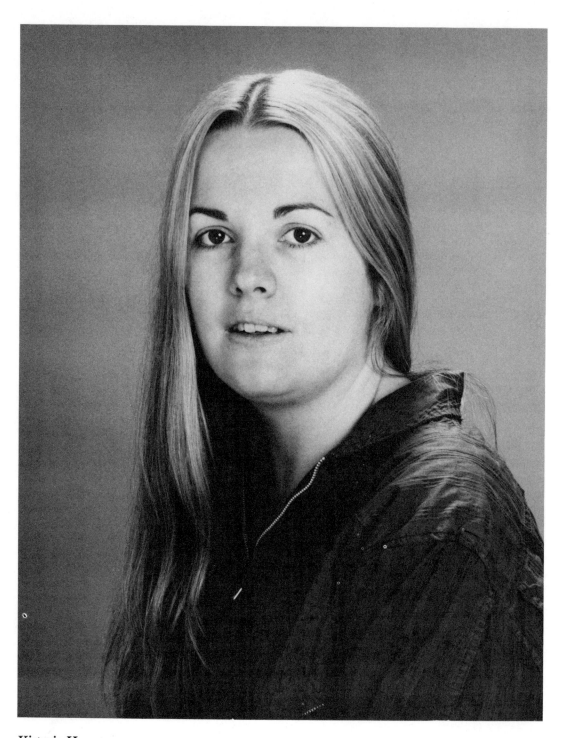

Victoria Hearst

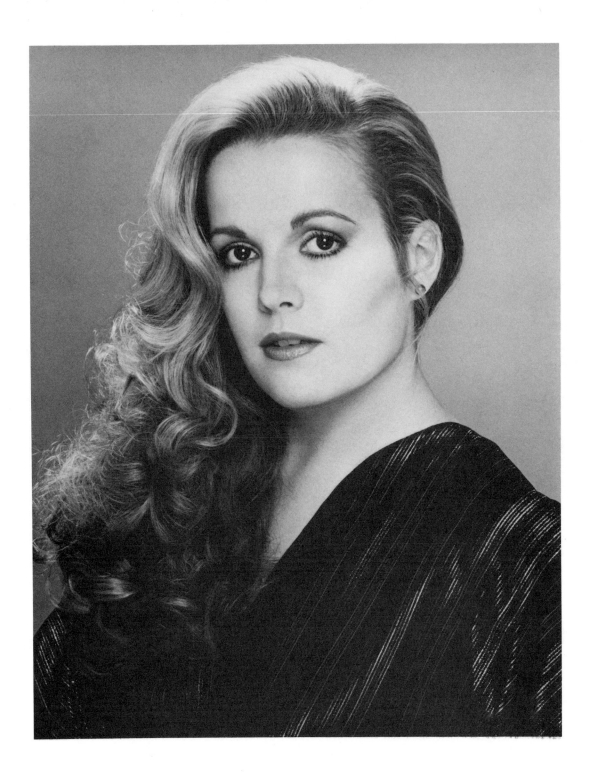

6. Translucent face powder.
7. Pink blusher on the "apple" of her cheeks.
7A. Neutral brown shadow on the sides of her nose to narrow it; highlighter down the center to make it look longer. (See optional Step 7A.)
8. Brown eye shadow in the crease of her lid; charcoal eye shadow at the outer corners and a light peach color on the eyelid; no inner eye liner; charcoal eye liner on top and bottom lids, smudged; two coats dark brown mascara.
9. No brow color; brows lightened one shade with highlight powder.
10. Lips lined with orange-brown lip liner extending slightly beyond her natural lip line; highlighter pencil to accent the crest of her upper lip; pale peach lipstick; lighter peach lipstick applied to the center of her lower lip to make it appear fuller; gloss.

FACE POWDER

Using just the tips of the sable bristles of your wide brush, dust translucent face powder all over your face. Stroke across your forehead, around the eyes, nose, mouth, and chin. Don't forget the eye sockets and neck.

Powder helps set the makeup and adds a nice matte finish. The powder should be translucent so that it doesn't interfere with the color of your foundation. Although baby powder is an excellent choice, my favorite is a

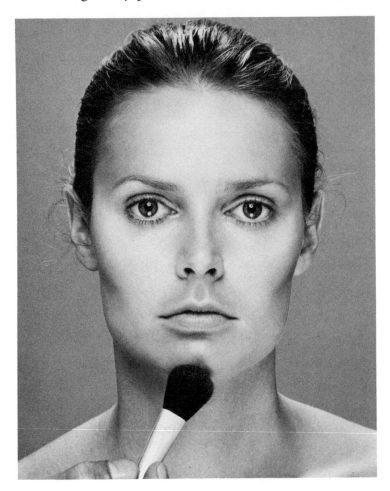

Step 6: Face powder

loose powder, Clubman, by Pinaud. This finely milled talc is available in beauty supply stores and costs about three dollars for eleven ounces—enough to last for a very long time. Since it's a professional product, it comes only in the large size, so transfer some of it to a small plastic shaker bottle. This way you can carry it with you for touch-ups during the day. If you prefer the convenience of a pressed powder compact, Lancôme's Maquifinish compact powder has a very silky texture.

I shake loose powder into the palm of my hand, dip the sable brush into it, and then flick off any excess before dusting the face. Use a minimal amount of powder, since too much can accentuate lines.

NASTASSIA KINSKI

NASTASSIA'S NATURAL FEATURES
Full face
Thick eyebrows
Large gray-green eyes
Full lips
Good jawline
Long neck

Nastassia Kinski almost never wears foundation—none for daytime unless it's required for photo sessions or films. She prefers the matte finish of translucent face powder. I used a very sheer liquid foundation and dusted her face frequently with loose powder to eliminate any trace of shine. In fact, she has a tiny scar on her left cheek which completely disppears when face powder is applied. Nastassia's skin tones are so even, her complexion so delicately textured, that she doesn't need the help of a foundation, and I would never recommend she use it for street wear.

This highly sensitive and emotional young actress has often been compared to some of the century's most beautiful women—Ingrid Bergman, Sophia Loren, Audrey Hepburn.

Nastassia says she finds it difficult to listen to comparisons of herself to some of the screen's greatest legends. "It is the most wonderful compliment, of course. But it is uncomfortable for me to be compared to these women."

However, the young star does not deny her own good looks. "There are times when I *feel* beautiful. I have become better looking as I have grown to be a better person. There was a time when I was bitter and confused, and it showed in my face. When a person is in love, they look the most beautiful. Or when a woman is pregnant. This is no coincidence. The love flows out and shows," she explains.

"My eyes are my best feature. If I could change something, it would be my behind," she states with a laugh. "Men like it, but I wish it were smaller and my chest were bigger."

Five-foot-eight Nastassia says, "I'm always extreme. I exercise for hours at a time and then not at all. I love ballet and can practice for hours. When I am not doing ballet, I work out at a health club."

The German-born actress is good to her skin, cleansing it religiously twice a day using products made by skin care expert Ole Henriksen. She faithfully applies moisturizer after each cleansing.

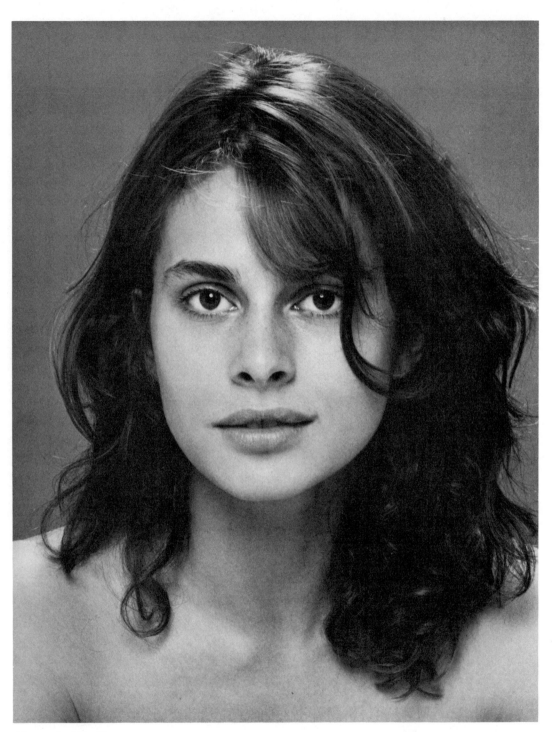

Nastassia Kinski

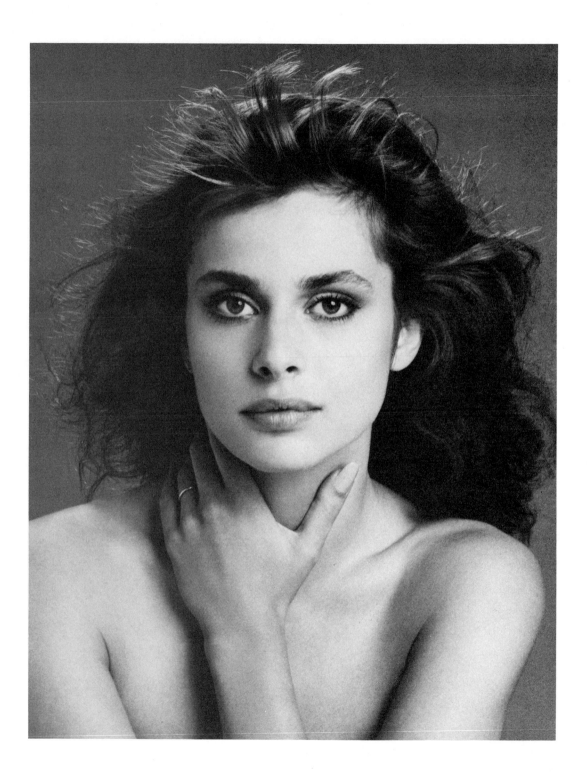

Even svelte Nastassia watches her weight, but she admits to some culinary passions: "Fruit, spaghetti, and chocolate cakes—but that is not to say they are all good for me."

Nastassia's Makeup

1. No blemish cover.
2. No concealer.
3. A very sheer, pale ivory liquid foundation, used only for photographs.
4. Highlighter above her cheekbones.
5. A little contour shadow (I prefer to emphasize the roundness of her face).
6. Translucent face powder to create a very matte finish, also reapplied at conclusion of makeup process.
7. Peach blusher on the "apple" of her cheeks and on her chin.
8. Charcoal gray eye shadow in the crease of the lid and more intense in the outer corners; brown shadow blended from the crease to the brow bone; no shadow on the lid; black inner eye liner on the upper lid, with light pink inner eye liner on the lower lid to make the eyes look even larger; charcoal eye liner smudged at the outer corners of both her upper and lower lids; black mascara.
9. No brow color; brows brushed up to emphasize their fullness.
10. No lip liner; coral lipstick; no gloss.

BLUSHER

Smile. Find the fullest part—or the "apple"—of your cheek. With your large sable brush, apply powder blusher on the "apple"—just between the highlighter and above the contour shadow. Avoid blending blusher directly under the eye. With the brush, blend upward and outward toward the ears, but do not blend higher than the top of the ear or lower than the ear lobes. Blend until color fades into the hairline. Use a cotton ball to continue blending the blusher until you have achieved a delicate, natural-looking glow. Blusher should always be used subtly.

One of the questions I hear most often is, Exactly where does my blusher go? If you follow the instructions above, you won't go wrong.

There are a few other spots that can use a touch of blusher, however. I often apply blusher to the temple area in order to tie in the color to the top of the face. If your forehead is very high, apply the blusher just under the hairline in the center of the forehead and blend. Apply a hint of blusher to the bridge of the nose (but not to the tip), because this is where the natural light of the sun would fall. A touch of blusher on the center of the chin can also add more color to the face. When wearing a low neckline, you might like a bit of blusher on the sides of the neck and in the cleavage. A touch of blusher on each earlobe can make a narrow face appear wider.

The color of the blusher you use should be the one that's the closest in color to your natural blush. If your skin is olive or sallow, clear shades in the pink and red family are a perfect complement. For ruddy skin, coral or peach tones can help balance the redness. Bronze and earth tones as well as bright corals are marvelous on a tanned face. Clear red is perfect for most black skin, while dark brick shades create a more dramatic effect. For evening, I have even used purple blushers on black skin.

Experiment by mixing a few different shades together. Since natural skin tones are a variety of colors, I often use many different shades to create one beautiful overall effect.

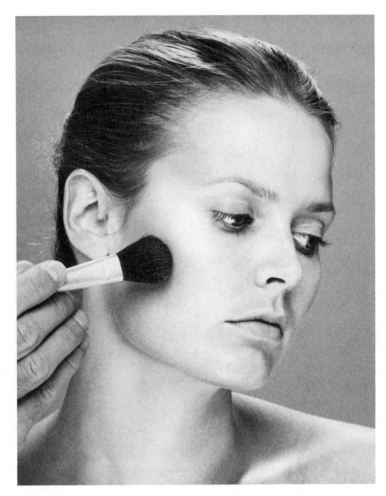

Step 7: Blusher

Indian Earth, an earth-toned powder sold in many department and health food stores, creates a subdued blush on almost any skin tone and is worth trying. Its soft and luminous effect works best when you're not wearing any foundation. Britt Ekland, who avoids the use of much color on her face, uses Indian Earth in the summer both as face makeup and as eye makeup to give her natural-looking tones.

Blusher, which used to be called rouge, is available in powder, cream, gel, and pencil form. I prefer the powder, but many women tell me that cream blushers last longer on their skin, especially if they have wrinkles or very dry skin. Cream blusher is worn in the same place as powder and is applied with the middle finger. I generally suggest that women with very oily skin avoid

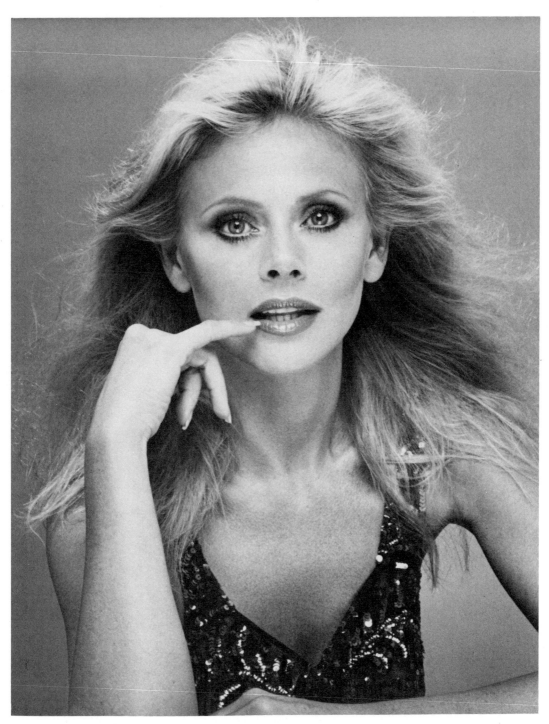

Britt Ekland (Hairstyle by Shannon McCullough)

cream blushers because the color seems to fade rapidly. However, some oily-skinned women have success by applying a cream blusher before applying face powder, and then dusting with a powder blusher.

When selecting a powder blusher, choose one that's smooth and silky. If it feels coarse and dry, it may streak and look chalky. Rub the blusher between your fingers as a test; if it feels the least bit coarse or grainy, try another. Try it on your face. It should blend nicely with your skin tone.

Gels create a translucent look but can have a drying effect on some complexions. That's why they're excellent for women with oily skin. Most blusher pencils are too difficult to apply and tend to pull the skin. I've used lipsticks as blusher, and they work very well. Some of the eye shadow shades sold in many beauty supply stores can be used as blushers, too. They're very inexpensive and come in a variety of pinks, reds, purples, and earth tones. Many blushers are frosted, producing a sheen. Normally, I shy away from products that are frosted, but they can have a very pleasant effect, particularly on dry skin, which often needs a little extra glow.

If your face is very angular and the hollows of your cheeks are very recessed, use blusher even more sparingly, only on the "apple" where you normally blush.

MORGAN BRITTANY

MORGAN'S NATURAL FEATURES
Widow's peak
Naturally dark, full brows
Wide-set, light blue eyes
Long lashes
Tiny bump on the bridge of her nose
Translucent pale complexion
Thin upper lip

Morgan Brittany's soft, ivory complexion gets a lift from blusher, since she tends to look a little pale without it. A soft rose blusher adds a delicate glow to her cheeks, chin, and temples.

"Perfume and cologne help create moods, and I take advantage of that. When I do a show, I match a perfume to the character, and that way, whenever I need it, the scent will remind me how to play the part." As the evil Kathryn Wentworth on "Dallas," Morgan wears Van Cleef and Arpels perfume.

It takes more than a sweet scent to achieve the success that Morgan has. She has worked hard and persisted and maintained a positive attitude. Despite being only five feet four inches tall, Morgan became one of the most sought-after cosmetics models in the business before landing her role on "Dallas." Her modeling career blossomed despite being told by the head of a major New York agency to lose ten pounds (she only weighed ninety-eight), get a nose job, and cut her hair. Morgan calmly closed her portfolio, said she was happy with her looks, and waved good-bye. Experiencing many similar rejections, she became even more determined, declaring, "I am going to do it!"—which, of course, she did.

To keep her complexion cover-girl clear, Morgan removes her makeup nightly with cold cream and then covers her face with a warm, steamy towel to open the pores. She goes over her face with a BufPuf (a sponge that removes dead skin cells) but uses no soap, which, she claims, dries her skin. Then she applies an astringent lotion and follows with eye cream and moisturizer. During the day she often spritzes her face with Evian mineral water (a light spray doesn't affect her makeup a bit) to give her skin a needed moisture boost. She rarely gets facials—once every six months at the most.

"I have a bump on the bridge of my nose, but photographers know how to minimize it with proper lighting," explains Morgan. "I've learned to live with it. As you get older,

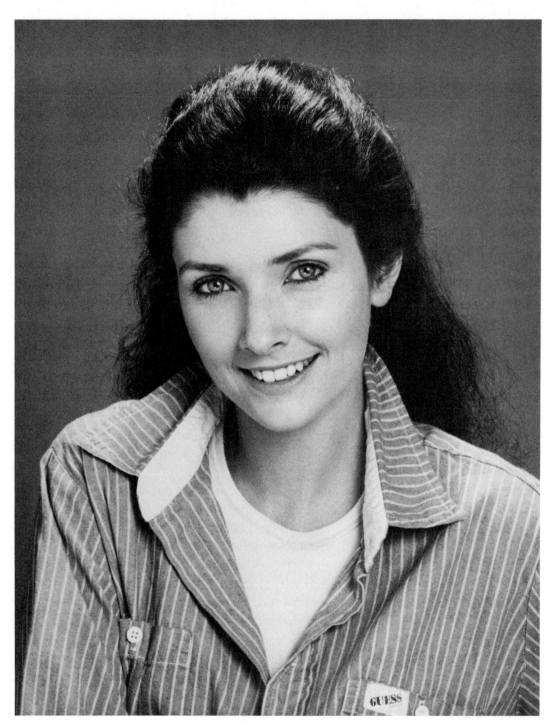

Morgan Brittany

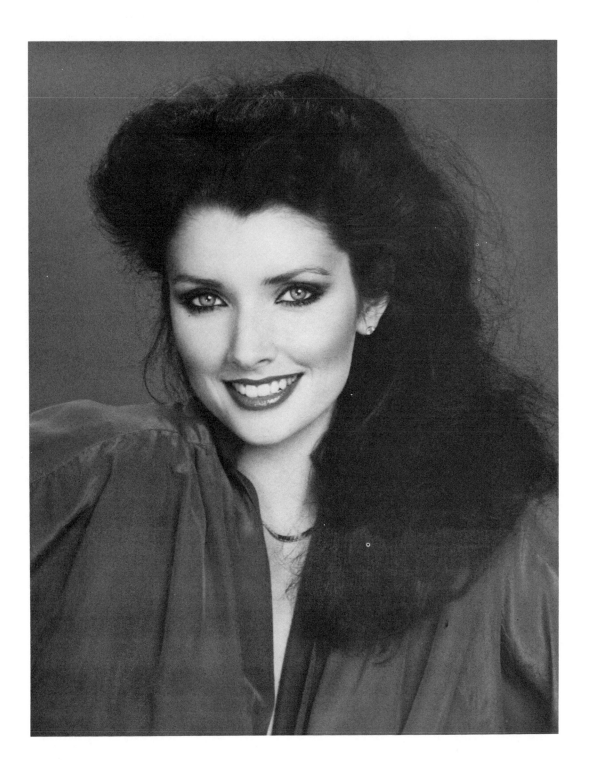

you realize that perfection is boring. I think it's better to let a flaw become part of your uniqueness."

—————————— Morgan's Makeup ——————————

1. No blemish cover.
2. No concealer.
3. Very light liquid foundation.
4. Highlighter above the cheekbones and immediately under the hollows of her cheeks.
5. Contour shadow at the temples to narrow her broad forehead and in the hollows of her cheeks to accent them.
6. Translucent face powder.
7. Rose blusher on cheeks, temples, and chin.
7A. A neutral brown shadow on the bump on her nose to minimize it.
8. Pinkish lavender eye shadow in the crease of the lid, extending out and upward to create a catlike look; light lavender shadow on the lid; black inner eye liner on top and bottom lids; muted purple eye liner on tops and bottoms; one coat of black mascara.
9. No brow color; brows brushed up.
10. Red lip liner, true red lipstick, and gloss—all to accent her gorgeous white teeth.

PEGGY FLEMING

PEGGY'S NATURAL FEATURES
Thick natural brows
Light blue green eyes with dark lashes
Discoloration around eyes
Some freckles
Natural recessed cheeks
Very high cheekbones

Olympic champion figure skater Peggy Fleming has a fair complexion with some yellow in it, so she uses blusher to brighten her face. With her fabulous high cheekbones and naturally hollow cheeks, she doesn't need contour shadow, so blusher helps to accentuate them, too. A dusting of blusher on her nose, chin, and forehead gives her a healthy, athletic glow.

Peggy has one of the loveliest complexions I've ever seen. She admits that she takes the best care of her skin when she is in a show, because then she wears heavy makeup, which requires more thorough cleansing. Since Peggy wears a great deal of eye makeup when she's working, she uses Chanel's Gentle Eye Makeup Remover to remove it after each show and then washes her face carefully with Neutrogena soap and a BufPuf to make sure that every trace of makeup is gone. She has never had a facial, rarely uses a moisturizer, and avoids the sun as much as possible.

Always the athletic type, Peggy has never had a weight problem. "That's because I watch what I eat and I'm active. I always eat half of what other people are eating, and if I have dessert one day, I skip it the next. I eat more fish and chicken than red meat."

She keeps her shiny brown hair long because she likes the way it flows when she skates. Although she's tried perming it, the treatment was too drying. She washes her hair every day with Mastey shampoo and conditioner. Hugh York styled Peggy's hair using large hot rollers. Then he back brushed it and styled it with his fingers.

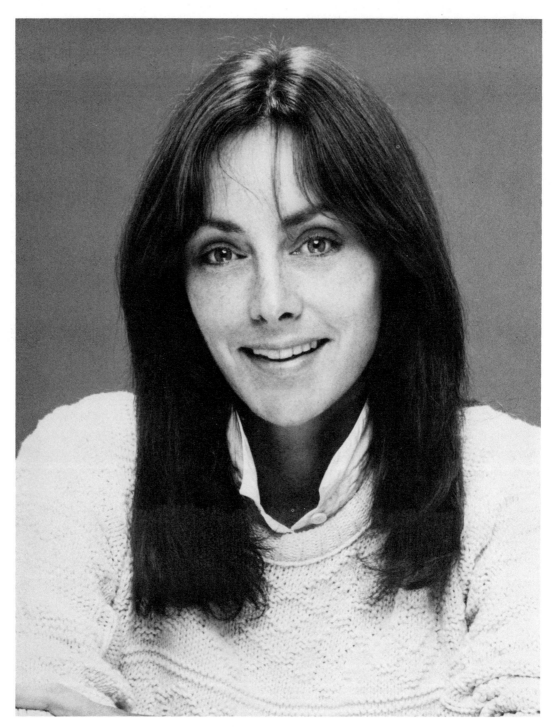

Peggy Fleming

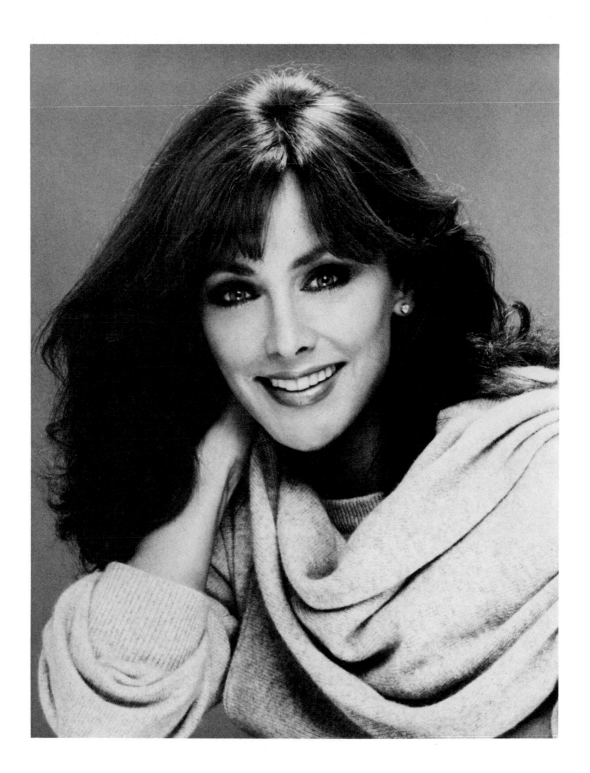

1. No blemish cover.
2. Concealer around the eyes.
3. Pinkish beige liquid foundation to even out her freckles.
4. Just a touch of highlighter above her naturally high cheekbones to accent them.
5. No contour shadow.
6. Translucent face powder.
7. Coral blusher on her cheekbones.
8. Smoky gray eye shadow in the crease of the lid; smoky gray shadow on the lid; no shadow on brow bone; black inner eye liner top and bottom; black outer eye liner top and bottom; two coats of black mascara.
9. No eyebrow pencil.
10. Reddish brown lip liner; reddish brown lipstick; gloss.

JANINE TURNER

JANINE'S NATURAL FEATURES
Even, pale complexion
Thick brows
Long lashes
Large green eyes
Upper lip slightly full

Janine Turner's alabaster complexion needs a delicate dusting of clear pink blusher to bring out her cheeks and to create a delicate glow. I put blusher not only on her cheeks, but also on her brow bone, forehead, and ear lobes, to add just a touch of color.

Best known as Laura on TV's "General Hospital," five-foot-six-and-a-half-inch Janine takes jazz dancing classes twice a week to keep in shape. She never misses her daily dosage of vitamin pills and wouldn't think of skipping her morning egg. She drinks water with the juice of one lemon in it to help cleanse her system and keep her skin clear. If she wakes up with swollen eyes, she puts two cold wet teabags on them and goes back to bed for ten minutes to contemplate her day.

Since television work demands that she wear heavy makeup, she is meticulous about cleaning her skin. Janine uses Revlon's herbal cleansing grains on a regular basis and a BufPuf to slough off dry skin cells. When she is troubled by oily skin, she uses Helena Rubenstein's clay cleanser. Rather than using astringents, Janine opts for cold water or a bit of alcohol. Though she is inconsistent about using a daytime moisturizer, she uses a night cream at bedtime. She also slathers her hands in night cream and slips on a pair of cotton gloves before turning out the light. Her soft hands are proof-positive that the regimen works.

After setting her hair in hot rollers, stylist Bruce Johnson brushed out Janine's hair creating a natural and sexy look.

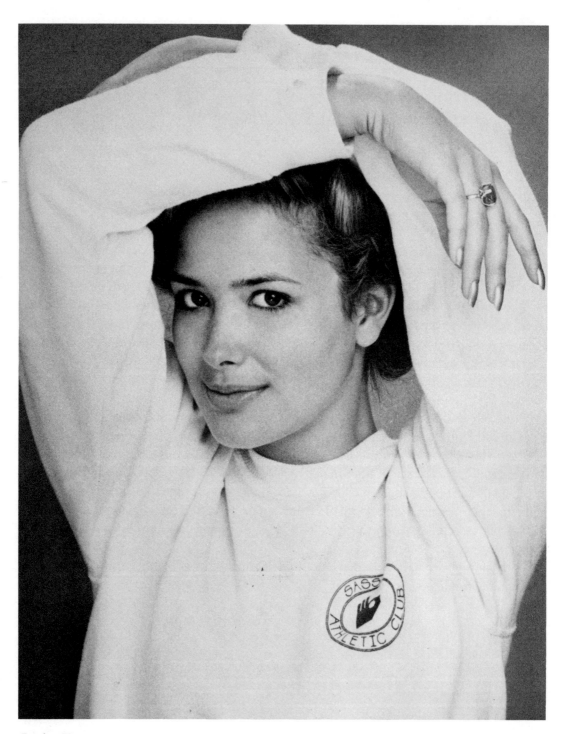

Janine Turner

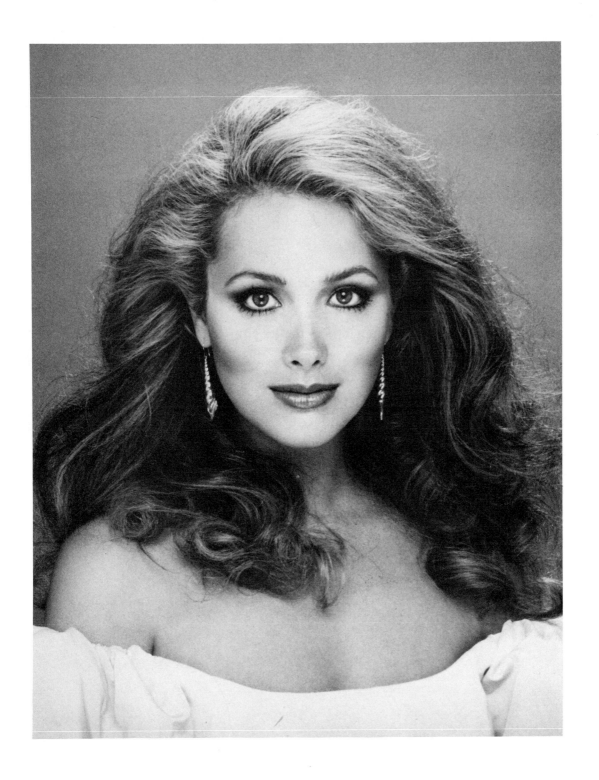

1. No blemish cover.
2. No concealer.
3. No foundation.
4. Highlighter above her naturally high cheekbones.
5. Contour shadow in the hollows of her cheeks and at the temples.
6. Translucent face powder.
7. Clear pink blusher on the cheeks, temples, chin, and bridge of her nose adds a delicate glow to her flawless skin.
8. Pinkish lavender eye shadow in the crease of the lid, extending from the inner corners to the outer triangle area; lavender shadow on the lids; black inner eye liner on upper lid only; muted purple eye liner on upper and lower lids, smudged slightly at the outer corners; one coat of black mascara.
9. Brows brushed up to accentuate their natural fullness.
10. Reddish purple lip liner slightly inside the natural lip line on the upper lip, while following the lip line on the lower lip; matching lipstick; gloss.

SHADING YOUR NOSE
(Optional)

If your nose appears wide, you may want to shade it, giving it a narrower or shorter appearance. This optional step is one I use often in photography but don't recommend too often for daytime wear. Some women become so adept at shading their noses, however, that they use the technique as a regular step in their evening makeup routine.

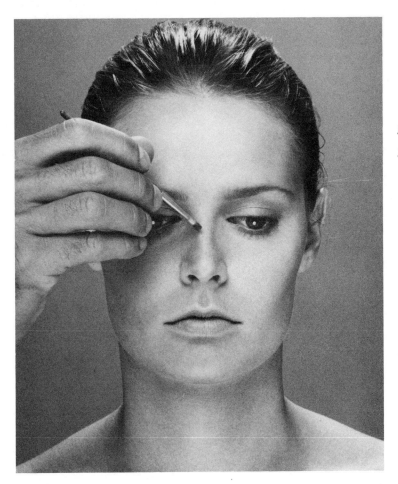

Step 7A: Shading your nose (optional)

I prefer using pressed powders to contour the nose—the application is easier to control. To highlight, use a shade approximately two shades lighter than your skin tone. Lancôme's Dual Finish Creme/Powder Makeup is easy to use. For shading, use a neutral gray brown shade such as On Stage's color called burlap.

Using a small sable brush, apply a narrow stripe of highlighter vertically from the bridge of the nose to the tip. With another small sable brush, shadow the sides of your nose with the neutral brown contour powder. Blend carefully with a cotton swab. Additional contour shadow can be used at the tip of the nose between the nostrils to create a shorter-looking nose. It can also be used on the sides of the nostrils to narrow a nose that is wide at the tip. Employ the utmost care when blending, or you may look like you have a dirty nose. This corrective step takes practice.

This step can also be used in the reverse, to widen a narrow nose. Use the contour shadow on the bridge of the nose and the highlighter along the sides.

MARY ANN MOBLEY

MARY ANN'S NATURAL FEATURES
Large brown eyes
Long lashes
Youthful, round cheeks
Olive skin with smooth texture
Tiny light freckles
Slightly wide nose
Full lips

Mary Ann Mobley looks gorgeous with or without makeup. But when she's photographed, her nose can look slightly wide, so I used shadow and highlighter to give it a slimmer illusion.

"I'm not tall—five feet four and a half inches—and I'm not the glamorous type at all," says this former Miss America. "In fact, I still remember thinking that someone was going to stop me as I was walking down the runway at the Miss America Pageant and say, 'Hey, little girl, we've made a mistake!'" Obviously, there was no mistake—her classic beauty and excellent figure proved that height doesn't matter.

"I hate to exercise, but I force myself to maintain a routine of body movements. I use the Pilates method, which concentrates on unifying mind and body, a technique that dancers use."

Mary Ann highlights her shoulder-length hair with subtle touches of blond and gold. For her after photo, Hugh York used hot rollers and a little back brushing for a loose, sexy hairstyle.

Her beauty routine is far more simple than her exercise regimen; it has to be, since her busy schedule as a housewife, mother, and career woman leaves little room for time-consuming regimens. "I don't like to spend too much time on myself. I want more out of life than how I look, what I wear, where I live, and what my next part will be. Giving and sharing are very important to me."

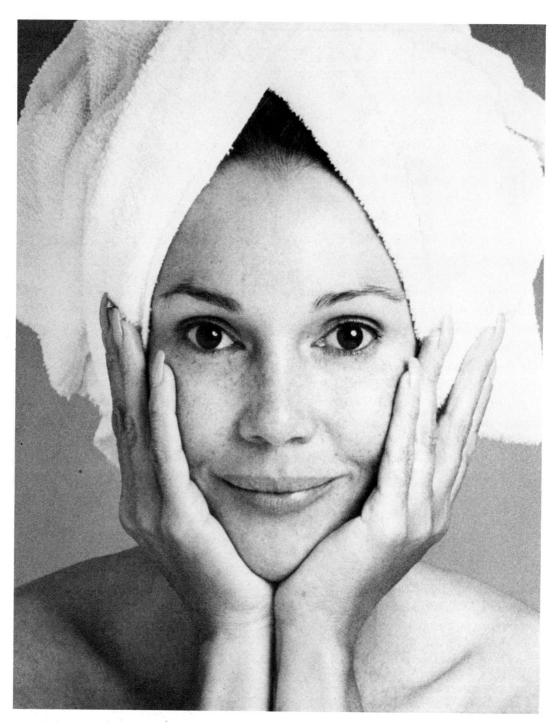

Mary Ann Mobley

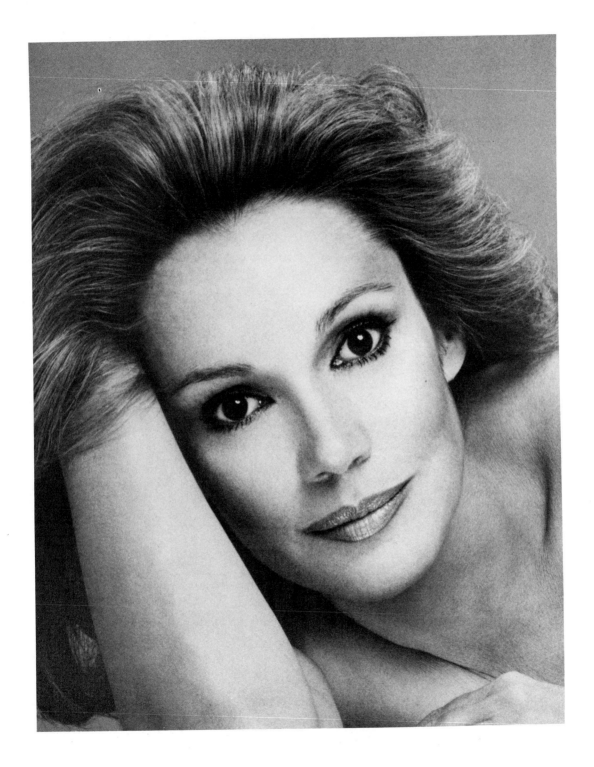

1. No blemish cover.
2. No concealer.
3. Medium beige foundation with pink undertones to balance her olive complexion.
4. Highlighter just above the cheekbones.
5. Contour shadow just below the cheekbones and on the temples.
6. Translucent face powder.
7. Clear pink blusher to accentuate her wonderful, full cheeks; a light touch of blusher on her chin and across the bridge of her nose for color.
7A. The sides of her nose are shaded with neutral brown contour shadow; highlighter is applied in a thin line from the bridge of the nose to the tip. All are carefully blended.
8. Rusty brown eye shadow at the crease of the lid and across the entire lid, blended up and out to the tip of the brow; charcoal shadow at outer corners blended into the rusty brown shadow; black inner eye liner on the upper lids; charcoal liner on the upper and lower lids, smudged slightly; black mascara.
9. Charcoal eyebrow pencil.
10. Pinkish red lipstick and lip liner; no gloss.

EYE MAKEUP

Using a small sable brush and pressed powder eye shadow, draw a thick line of shadow across the crease of your eyelid, starting at the inside corner and extending to the outer corner, and form a small triangle of shadow that points toward your temple (see photo A). Blend with your brush. Then, with a sharpened eye liner pencil, first line your lower lids, starting at the outside corner, along and just below the lash line, stopping the line in the center of your lower lid (see photo B). Smudge the line with your little finger or with a cotton swab. With the same pencil, line the entire upper lid, beginning at the inner corner of the eye and working toward the outer corner. Darken the triangle at the outer corner of the eye with additional eye liner pencil, then smudge (photo C). With a black eye liner pencil, line the upper inner lid (photo D). If your eyes are very small, you can make them appear larger by lining the lower inner lids with a white pencil (photo E). Using a small sable brush, apply color to the center of the lid (photo F). Using a sable brush, apply a small amount of shadow to the brow bone. Blend downward toward the crease shadow (photo G). Curl the eyelashes. Apply two coats of brown or black mascara to both upper and lower lashes (photo H).

Even if they avoid other forms of cosmetics, most women tell me they wear some kind of eye makeup. Your eyes project your mood, express your thoughts, and can even indicate your state of health, so why not make them look as beautiful as possible?

The most frequent mistake women make is to match their eye shadow color to the color of their eyes. Eye shadow is used to call attention to your eyes, not to overpower them. Avoid bright green, blue, turquoise, or other very bright shades.

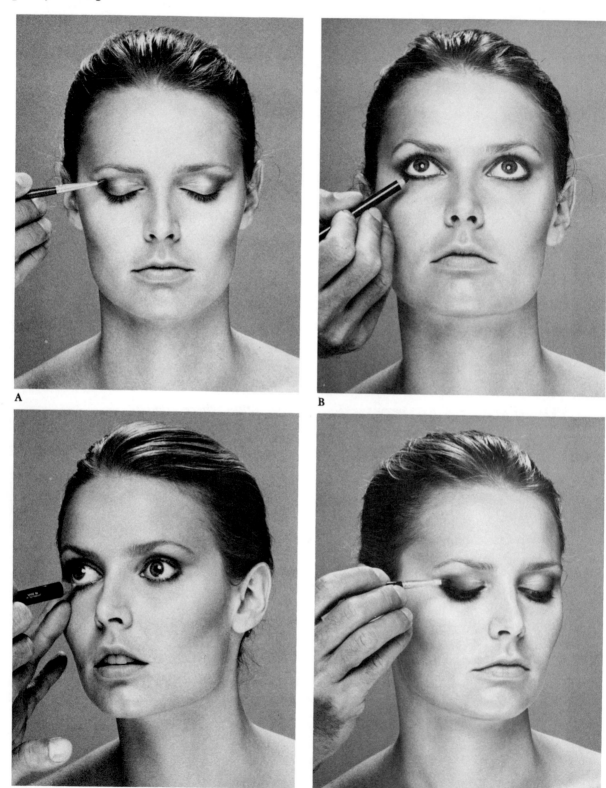

A

B

E

F

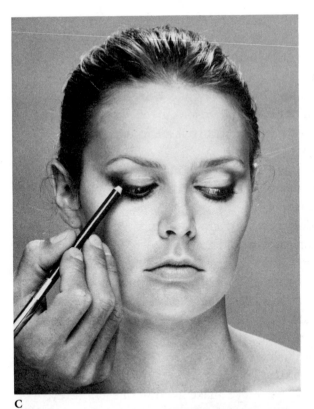

C

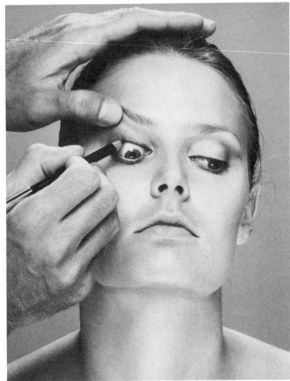

D

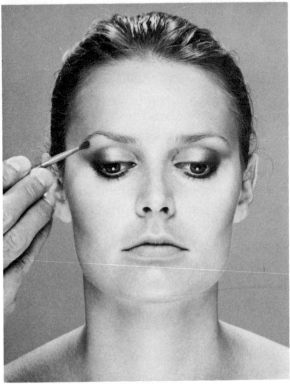

G

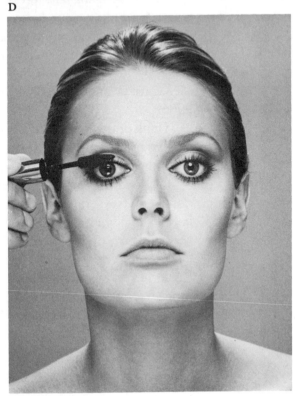

H

If you like shadows with a definite hue, opt for muted shades. Colorful shades can sometimes be effective if you wish to coordinate them to your outfit. Blue eyes can look very dramatic when shaded with slate blue (which is actually a muted gray with a blue undertone), reddish brown, lavender, or tan. Brown eyes can wear almost any shade. Plum or lavender not only look lovely with green eyes, they actually tend to make the eyes look greener. Muted blues and navy are excellent for green or hazel eyes as well. Slate blue shadow is particularly flattering to women with gray hair.

Remember, there are no hard and fast rules about what colors you're *supposed* to wear. Experiment, but always make certain that *the color of your eyes* is more prominent than the eye shadow.

I prefer pressed powder shadow because I find it so easy to use. Cream shadow can be easier to apply on dry or wrinkled skin, but powdered color still works as well. You can find all the shades you'll need on those revolving racks in the supermarket, dime store, or drug store. Revlon's Super Rich Colorcreme Eyeshadow goes on smoothly and evenly and comes in a huge array of colors, including a wonderful slate blue. Just make sure that your powder shadows don't dry out. A powder that's too dry can irritate the skin and can be difficult to blend. For the most natural look, avoid any frosted shadows during the day, particularly if you have wrinkled lids.

Before applying any pressed powder eye makeup, dust the entire eye region, including your lashes and brows, with face powder, so your eye shadow won't streak and your lash and brow color will last longer. Actually, I use rice powder in the eye area. This fine, dry powder is the perfect base for eye makeup. Find it in markets that specialize in Chinese imports or write to Paula McKenna, Vanity Inc., 704 North La Cienega, Los Angeles, California 90069.

Think of the eye area as being divided into three parts: the lid, the crease, and the brow bone. The crease separates the lid from the brow bone. It folds when the eye opens, so it can take the most intense color.

I always begin by shading the crease (photo A), thereby defining the shape of the eye. Next comes eye liner (photo B). Since I usually want to soften the line by smudging it, I always use eye color pencils or crayons, the most versatile form of eye makeup. Pencils should be soft so they don't pull the tender skin of your eyelids. Test the pencils in the store—if they drag on your hand, they'll drag on your lid. Layla pencils, which are carried in many beauty supply stores, are excellent and reasonably priced. Pressed powder liner can also be used, with a very small brush, but excess powder often dots the skin with hard-to-remove little black flecks. Cake eyeliner is easy to use but difficult to smudge.

To be successful with eye liner pencils and crayons, sharpen them frequently. Buy a sharpener with two holes, one for a regular-sized pencil and another for a wider crayon. Also, freeze your pencils before attempting to sharpen them. Freezing hardens the colored lead and allows you a more precise point. If your pencils get hard with age, run the tip under hot water for a few minutes, or hold the tip between your fingers so that the heat generated softens it.

When you draw the line on your lower lid, never extend the eye liner to the inside corner of your eye—unless your eyes are extremely wide set. Don't be afraid to apply the liner a little heavier at the outside corner of the eye. After you smudge it, this extra color will make your eyes appear larger. In most cases, eye liner on your upper lid should be the same color as the liner on the lower lid. Be sure to smudge it well to avoid a harsh line.

Women with close-set eyes should only line the outer half of each eye. Small eyes tend to look smaller when heavily lined. If your eyes droop downward, slant the upper eye liner up ever so slightly at the outer corners of the eye.

Charcoal gray is an excellent color choice for eye liner, particularly for daytime. Brunettes can wear black eye liner during the day if it is smudged and blended well, but brown shades can give a softer look. Muted purple shades work well for day or evening, especially if you incorporate the same shades in your lid shadow. Navy liner complements muted purple, charcoal, and slate blue shadows.

Inner eye liner, as shown in photos D and E, defines the eye. Gently lift the lid with one hand to expose the inside rim of the eye. Use the other hand to line the upper inner lid, under the lashes, from the outside corner to the inside corner. This defines the eye. I apply black inner liner to the upper lid on most women (except those with close-set eyes) no matter what color their eyes or hair might be.

Unless you have extremely large or protruding eyes, it's not a good idea to use black liner on the lower inner lid—it can make your eyes look smaller. Instead, choose a white eye liner pencil to create the illusion of a larger white area. Tired, red eyes will look brighter if you use a light blue lower inner liner. A blue pencil can also be flattering to blue eyes, as long as the shade is very subtle. A light green pencil used on the lower inner lid will flatter green or gray green eyes. Light lavender or pink inner liner will also complement green eyes.

An important note: If you wear contact lenses, do *not* use inner eye liner.

Once you have defined the shape of your eye with crease shadow and eye liners, it's time to add a touch of color. Remember that the primary intent of eye shadow is to enhance your *eyes,* not to draw attention to your clothing.

Although your eyes may appear brown, blue, or green, the iris is actually composed of dozens of specks of color. Look closely in a mirror and you may discover a rainbow you never knew existed. Many brown eyes have traces of green, black, red, and yellow. Blue or green eyes may also be flecked with lavender, purple, and gray. To highlight these intricate natural blends of color, I often combine two or three shades of shadow, selecting colors I actually see in the eye. I might use brown and green or pink and lavender on a blue eye, or green and slate blue on a brown eye. Although I usually avoid green shadow on green eyes and blue shadow on blue eyes, brown-eyed women can wear any shade. Try combining colors from the same family on the three areas on the eye. For example, brown in the crease, tan on the lid, and peach on the brow bone. The colors must be blended so there's no obvious line between them. Experimentation is fun, especially when you keep in mind that the only disaster is too much color. Blending and smudging with your fingertip or with a cotton swab will keep your eye shadow color soft and subtle.

Before applying color to your lid, stroke the brush across your hand to blot excess powder. Apply the color to the center of the lid and blend across the entire lid, concentrating most of the color on the outer corner at the "triangle" (see photo F). If additional color is desired, reapply and blend, always brushing the first stroke across your hand to eliminate excess powder, which may cause streaks.

For deep-set eyes, use a very light shadow on the entire lid, blending into the triangle area. For protruding eyes, shadow the entire lid with a medium to dark shade. For close-set eyes, apply a light shade from the center of the lid to the inside corner of the eye. For evening or low-light conditions, frosted eye shadow color can create a shimmery, flattering effect. If you choose frosted or iridescent loose powders, use a sponge-tipped applicator instead of a brush— the color goes on more smoothly.

When adding shadow to the brow bone (photo G), be sure the overall color is never more intense than the colors used on the lid area. Pale pink shadows look marvelous; so do peach and other muted pastels. Try using blusher on the brow bone; it creates a beautiful effect. A dark shadow on the brow bone can make the eyes look larger by creating the illusion of lifting the eye crease. If you have protruding eyes, a very light shade or highlighter on the brow bone will draw attention away from the lids, but never use white. It isn't always necessary to use eye shadow on the brow bone; never use so much that it detracts from the eye. If the eye area is wrinkled, the brow bone naturally appears lower and more prominent, so using highlighter would only accentuate this.

Curling eyelashes before applying mascara is a step that's too often overlooked. It helps to separate and lift the lashes, making the eyes seem larger and more alive. Tilt your head back, look down into a mirror, and clamp the curler as near as possible to the base of your lashes. Hold it closed for ten seconds. Release and clamp again, this time at the ends of the lashes. If you feel any pull on your lashes, the rubber insert in the curler may be soiled with old mascara or worn out. If so, replace it.

I only use three shades of mascara: brown, dark brown, and black. More often than not, I use black. Nature never provided green, blue, or purple lashes, so why would anyone use them where a natural look is called for? Blondes and redheads can achieve a very natural effect with brown or dark brown mascara, while brunettes can use black with the same results.

I like to use Lancôme's Immencils Gentle Lash Thickener, which is sold at most department stores. It's expensive compared to other brands, but it doesn't smudge, clump, or flake—a nice plus for contact lens wearers. Maybelline's Great Lash is also one of the best mascaras I've used, and it's priced very reasonably. Remember that mascara doesn't last forever. It may become dry. If your current supply is more than six months old, replace it.

If you prefer cream mascara to the wand type, try using a child's toothbrush to apply it. Ella Bache, a French cream mascara available at fine skin care salons, will keep your lashes from clumping. Cake mascara is also excellent for a very clean look. To prevent infection, never use saliva to moisten the cake (or any cosmetics product, for that matter). Use clean water or eye drops to form a smooth paste that can easily be stroked on the lashes.

To apply mascara (photo H), color your lower lashes first. Look down into a mirror and, holding the wand vertically, brush across the lashes with the point of the brush. Then, using the length of the brush, lightly separate the lashes. For the upper lashes, first coat the top of the lashes from base to tip, then the underside from base to tip. For thicker, darker lashes, apply a second coat. Another trick is to brush baby powder (or any translucent powder) on your lashes after the first coat before applying the second. If your newly colored lashes leave traces of wet mascara on the area just below your brows, try tilting your head back and looking down into your mirror while applying mascara to your upper lashes.

If your lashes are sparse or very short, artificial lashes can supplement what you've got. Ideally, they should be reserved for evening and should look as natural as possible. I prefer dark brown human hair lashes, although some synthetic lashes look fine if they are cut and fitted properly. Black lashes may look too artificial. My preference is for the individual lashes, but many women prefer the strips, which are applied along the base of the natural lashes. Either way, the entire process shouldn't take more than a few minutes.

Before applying the strip-style lashes, be sure to snip the length of the strip so that it exactly matches the length of your own lash line. If the strip is too stiff, you may have trouble applying it. To soften, place the lashes on a table and rub the strip for a few seconds with a blunt instrument, such as the handle of your scissors or the wooden tip of a makeup brush.

To apply, first position a hand mirror flat on a table so that you can conveniently look down into it. Next, apply clear surgical glue or lash adhesive to the base of the artificial lashes. (Never use colored glue or adhesive; the clear is best.) Looking down into the mirror, press the strip as close as possible to the base of your own lash line. After applying, make sure the ends of the strip are firmly in place. If they pop up, dot a bit of glue on each end of the strip and press down again.

If the lashes look too long when they're firmly in place, carefully trim them, using manicure scissors. The longest lashes should be in the center, not on the outside corner. Check the length from the front and side, making sure they look as natural as possible. Also look down into the mirror to check that the strip is applied evenly. If you wish to use artificial lower lashes, they may be applied in the same way.

Artificial eye lashes that are applied individually tend to look more natural than the strip type. Cut the strip into tiny sections with just a few hairs in each section. Using tweezers, pick up the sections one at a time, dab with adhesive, and wait a moment to allow the glue to become sticky. Apply the shortest lashes where your own are shortest and the longest toward the center of your lash line. Again check a mirror for symmetry and trim if necessary.

Always apply mascara *after* the artificial lashes are secured.

To remove strip lashes, peel off the lashes very gently. Be careful not to remove your own real lashes with them. An oily makeup remover will help soften the adhesive.

SHIRLEY JONES

SHIRLEY'S NATURAL FEATURES
Clear, smooth skin
Round cheeks
Round, dark blue eyes
Eyes slant downward
Long, light lashes
Ample space between eyes and brows
Nose wide at the tip

Shirley Jones has had the same perky young look for the last fifteen years. She's amazing. Her eyes, which have a naturally exaggerated crease and tend to slant downward slightly at the outer corners, get a lift from eye liner and from shadow in the outer corners. Extending the outer triangle of color upward lifts the eye.

With her ageless face and her childlike spirit, Shirley says, "I never think about growing older. As long as you're healthy and active, that's all there is to it. I think young; I feel young. I spend a great deal of time in the outdoors, because fresh air makes me feel vital. I ski when I can and I walk every chance I get."

Shirley has kept her hair short for the last fifteen years. "I don't like to have hair around my face. I look fine in hats and turbans because they pull the hair back and let my features show." For the photo shown here, hairstylist Barron used a curling iron to create a soft pixie look for Shirley's pretty, short hair. Shirley says she's always felt pretty but not beautiful. "I'm not too thrilled with my nose—never have been. It looks like a little crab apple sitting on a face. And my cheekbones should be higher and sharper. But basically I like my face—it's me."

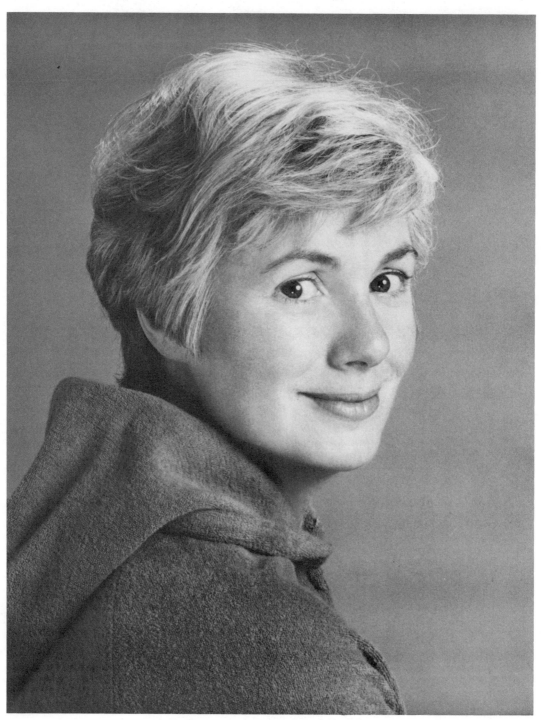

Shirley Jones

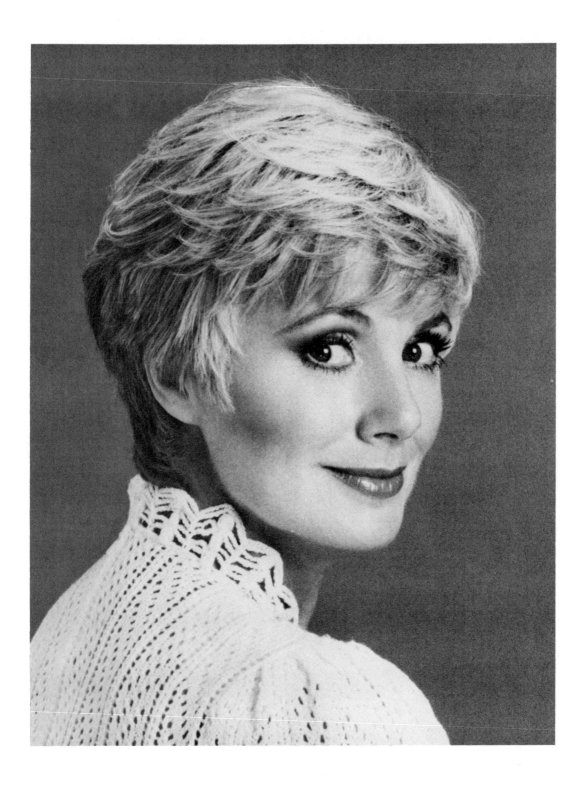

1. No blemish cover.
2. A bit of concealer under the eyes.
3. Beige liquid foundation.
4. Highlighter above the cheekbones.
5. Contour shadow below the cheekbones to define and slim her face.
6. Translucent face powder.
7. Slightly iridescent peach blusher on the "apple" of her cheeks.
7A. Neutral brown contour shadow on the sides of her nose to slim it slightly, and highlighter from the bridge to the tip to lengthen it.
8. Medium brown eye shadow to further define her pronounced crease; peach shadow on the lid and brow bone; black inner eye liner on the top lid only; charcoal eye liner on the top and bottom lids, slightly smudged; one coat of black mascara on her naturally long lashes.
9. No eyebrow pencil; brows brushed up for fullness.
10. Orange-brown lip liner; pale orange-brown lipstick; gloss.

CONNIE SELLECCA

CONNIE'S NATURAL FEATURES
Thick, natural brows
Magnificent green eyes
Dark lashes
Flawless olive skin
High cheekbones
Face that can appear too narrow at times
Full lips

Connie Sellecca's green eyes are one of her best features, so I don't need to add too much color around them—I want their natural color to stand out. I used neutral smoky shades on her lids and no shadow at all in the crease. That's an unconventional technique for me, but I wanted nothing to detract from the intense green of her beautiful eyes. Black eye liner on both the inner and outer lids, together with black mascara, accentuated her green eyes perfectly.

Throughout her pregnancy, Connie, who played a lawyer on TV's "The Greatest American Hero," maintained a rigorous schedule of working and exercising to keep herself in top form. "I was in the best shape ever. I was eating properly and working out religiously three times a week at Jane Fonda's Studio, where they have special classes for pregnant women. My skin and hair looked better than they had in years." She gained forty-seven pounds with the pregnancy, but within six months after Gib's birth, she had dropped fifty-one pounds. The five-foot-eight-inch brunette now weighs 115.

Connie lifts weights and does body-building routines to create a few more curves on her lean frame. "What would I change about myself? I wish I had better legs and a more shapely rear end."

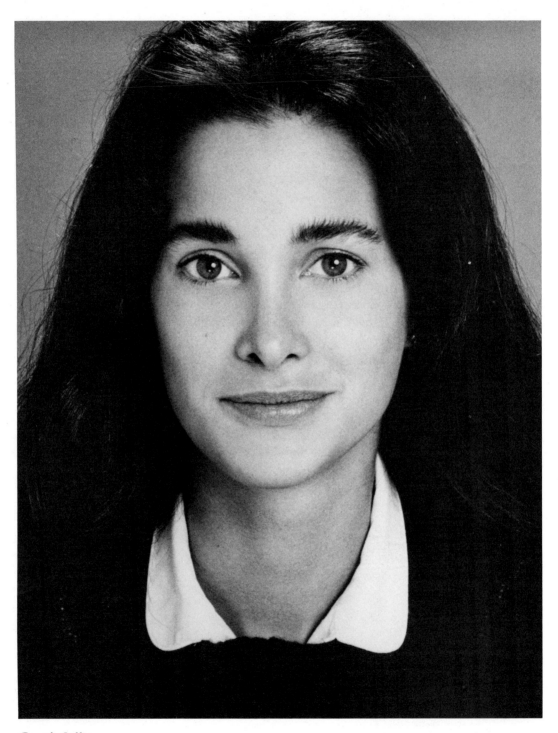

Connie Sellecca

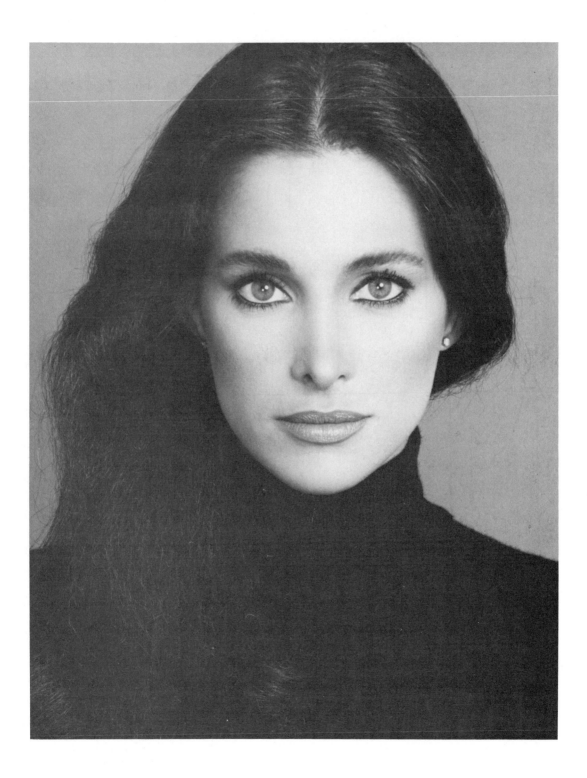

1. No blemish cover.
2. No concealer.
3. Medium beige liquid foundation.
4. Highlighter above the cheekbones.
5. Contour shadow to create the illusion of hollows in her cheeks.
6. Translucent face powder.
7. Muted coral blusher on the cheekbones.
7A. Highlighter along the sides of her nose to diminish its vertical line.
8. No eye shadow in the crease of the lid; charcoal on the lid; none on the brow bone; black inner eye liner on top and bottom lids; black outer eye liner on top and bottom; two coats of black mascara.
9. No eyebrow pencil; brows brushed up.
10. Brown lip liner; rusty beige lipstick; no gloss.

JESSICA WALTER

JESSICA'S NATURAL FEATURES
Low forehead
Nicely spaced dark brown eyes
Good bone structure
Dimples
Clear, light olive complexion
Large mouth
Long neck

Jessica Walter's eyes are so expressive that I used dark shadows and liners, blended and smudged, to make them look even darker and somewhat mysterious.

Perhaps best known for her role in the film *Play Misty for Me* and as the vicious Ava on NBC's "Bare Essence," Jessica showed what a fine actress she is—off camera she couldn't be sweeter. Her warmth shows immediately in her sincere smile and in her intense eyes. Jessica shares my attitude about beauty: "Everybody's unique. Take advantage of what's special about you, and don't try to be like everybody else."

Since Jessica has coarse, thick hair, she keeps it layered so she can wear it very casually. A few short, soft bangs camouflage her low forehead and give her hairstyle a fresh look.

Although she considers herself to be five years behind in fashion, she always looks very chic. Since she never has had a weight problem, Jessica looks terrific in the jeans she usually wears during the day. She swims daily to keep in top shape and avoids butter, oils, fried foods, and meat in order to keep her body healthy inside and out.

Jessica's Makeup

1. No blemish cover.
2. No concealer.
3. Medium beige foundation with a hint of pink in it to balance the sallowness in her olive complexion.
4. Highlighter above her cheekbones.
5. Contour shadow below her cheekbones.
6. Translucent face powder.

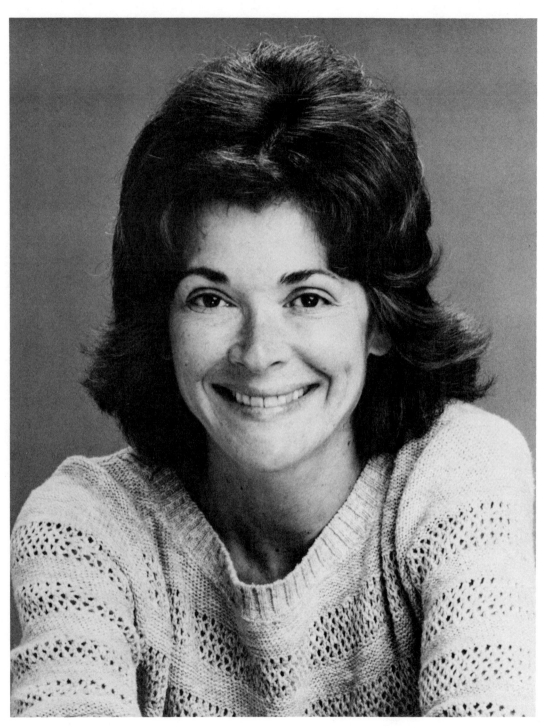

Jessica Walter

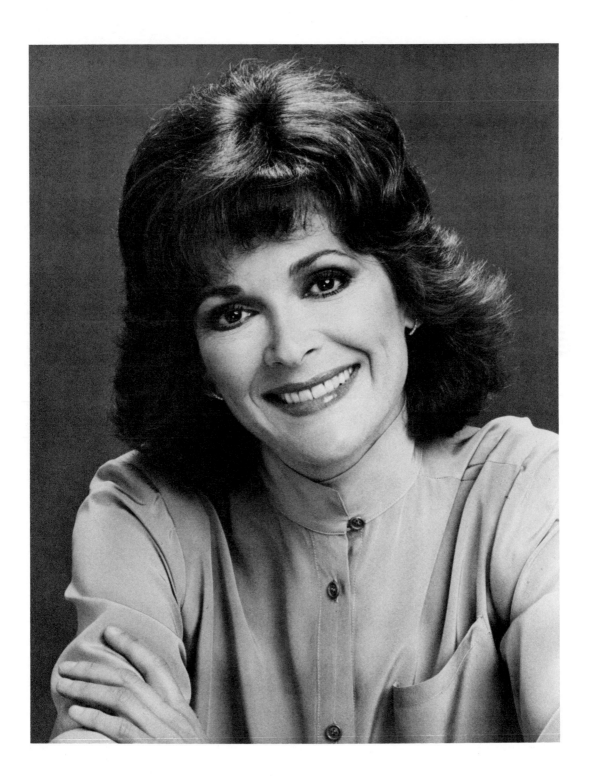

7. Reddish brown blusher on her cheekbones.
8. Reddish brown eye shadow on the crease and on the lid, blending up toward the brow; charcoal shadow at the outer corners, blended into the shadow at the crease; black inner liner on the upper lids; black liner on the upper and lower lids, slightly smudged to create a smoky look; two coats of black mascara.
9. Brows brushed with a beige-tint powder to lighten them slightly.
10. Reddish brown lip liner; slightly lighter reddish brown lipstick; gloss.

EYEBROWS

Brush brows upward with an eyebrow brush or with a child's toothbrush. Apply eyebrow pencil (photo A) with short strokes in the same direction in which the hair grows. Always use a light hand; never pull the skin. Blend with your finger or with a cotton swab.

Eyebrow pencil should look very natural and can help to offset your beautiful eyes. Choose a pencil soft enough to go on smoothly but not one that is as soft as eye liner pencils. Maybelline's Brow & Liner Pencil is great and inexpensive.

A

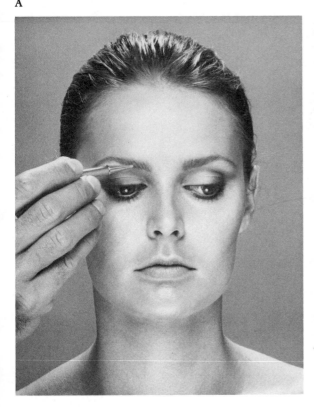

B

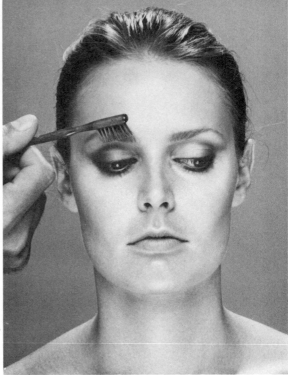

Step 9: Eyebrows

The color should match your brow's natural shade, unless your brows are so light that they don't show. If that's the case, choose pencils slightly darker than your brows. Use two or more pencils in different shades to achieve a natural effect. For light brows, use a light brown or silvery beige or a combination of both. If you're a redhead, try light brown and a hint of auburn—but be careful: Too much auburn looks orange and artificial. Not even the darkest brunettes should use pure black on dark brows. Instead, try dark brown or charcoal or a combination of both.

If your brows are too dark and you don't want to bleach them, try using a bit of foundation on them to lighten them slightly. Highlighter powder also works well as a temporary lightener.

Pencils should always be soft but sharp. I like the retractable eyebrow pencils made by Revlon and Max Factor. They're like drafting pencils and always stay sharp.

After coloring, brush your eyebrows upward to further blend the pencil and to make the brows look fuller. If they're stubborn, keep them in place with a liquid fixative called Perma-Brow, found at many beauty supply stores. Don't get it on the skin around your brows, as it has a tendency to shine. Another technique is to spray your eyebrow brush with hair spray or coat it with a dab of moustache wax or ordinary hand soap before brushing.

MARCIA LOWRY

MARCIA'S NATURAL FEATURES
Low brow bone
Short brows
Wide-set light blue eyes
Thin lips
Large mouth
Good jawline
Wide face

When I first looked at Marcia Lowry's face, I saw two dark dashes over her pretty blue eyes. With such heavy, short brows near the center of her face, her eyes appeared to be closer-set than they actually are. I suggested that we lighten her brows one shade and extend them with brow pencil to achieve a more natural look.

An executive in the advertising industry, Marcia had never worn makeup before she came to see me. She wanted to give her husband a special gift; and what could be more special, she thought, than a photograph of a sexy new version of herself. I suggested that Marcia let her hair grow longer and get a perm before we took her after photo. And we talked about makeup routines and a regimen that she could easily incorporate into her life.

Months later, dressed in a luxurious black mink coat, Marcia posed for the photo. Delighted with the results, she inscribed the gift, "What becomes a legend most? Marcia!"

Her husband's reaction? "He was shocked at first, but not anymore. Now I wear makeup to work every day. I know a good thing when I see it."

Marcia's Makeup

1. No blemish cover.
2. No concealer.
3. Beige cream foundation to cover freckles.
4. Highlighter above cheekbones.
5. Contour shadow below the cheekbones, blended into her jawline to slim her face.

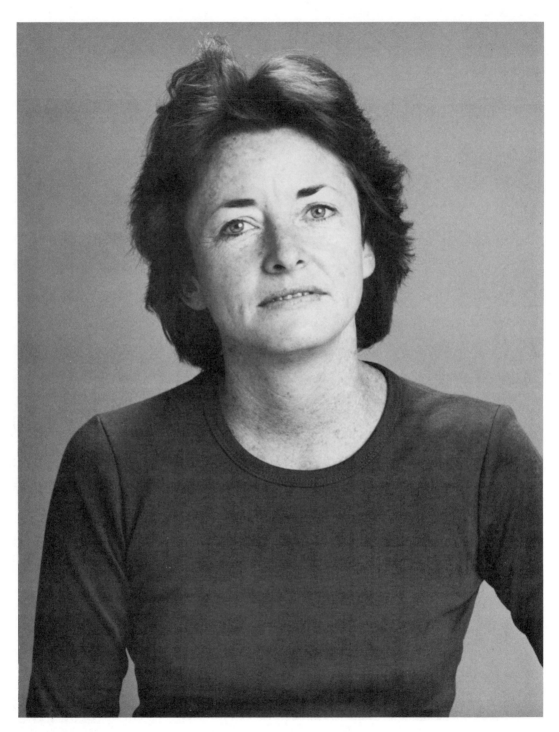

Marcia Lowry

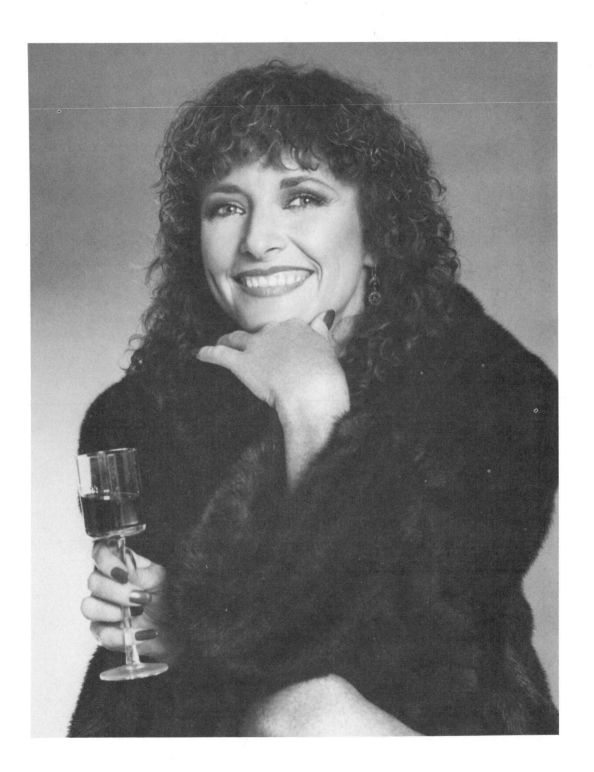

6. Translucent face powder.
7. Rose blusher on the cheeks.
8. Plum eye shadow on the crease of the lid, blended up toward the brow; lavender shadow on the lids; black inner eye liner on top and bottom lids; charcoal eye liner on upper and lower lids, smudged slightly at corners; two coats of black mascara.
9. Brown eyebrow pencil to extend the length of her brows and to increase their fullness.
10. Reddish purple lip liner slightly outside the natural lip line to create fuller lips; reddish purple lipstick; gloss.

MARGAUX MIRKIN

MARGAUX'S NATURAL FEATURES
No eyebrows
Pale, flawless skin
Lots of eyelid
Beautiful, large light brown eyes
Eyes droop a bit at corners
Flat cheekbones, oblong face
Long neck
Full lips
Slightly receding chin

Margaux Mirkin doesn't have any eyebrows—they simply never grew in. I suggested she pencil in light, natural-looking brows to frame her heavy-lidded eyes, retaining a romantic, feminine look.

Margaux grew up in the world of high finance, so it's no surprise that she grew up to become an entrepreneur. But Margaux didn't take the "budget" route; she opted for luxury, establishing a car rental business she calls Drive-A-Dream. She has her own collection of twenty-five exotic cars, which she stores in climate-controlled garages behind her Los Angeles home.

Margaux meticulously cares for her pale ivory skin with Clinique products and exercises regularly to keep her five-foot-seven-inch body at its slimmest. She runs six and a half miles daily and practices ballet four times a week.

Margaux's Makeup

1. No blemish cover.
2. No concealer.
3. Very pale beige, matte-finish liquid foundation.
4. Highlighter above her cheekbones and at the center of her chin.
5. Contour shadow applied low under the cheekbones to avoid narrowing her face.
6. Translucent face powder.
7. Muted coral blusher.

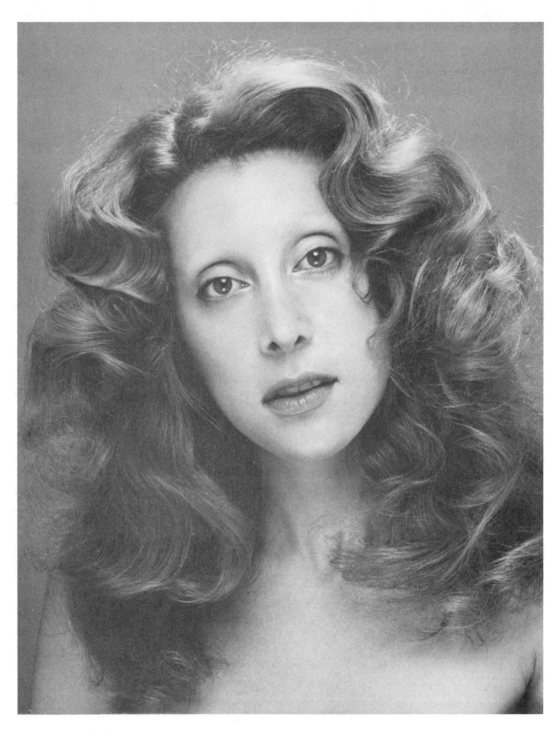

Margaux Mirkin

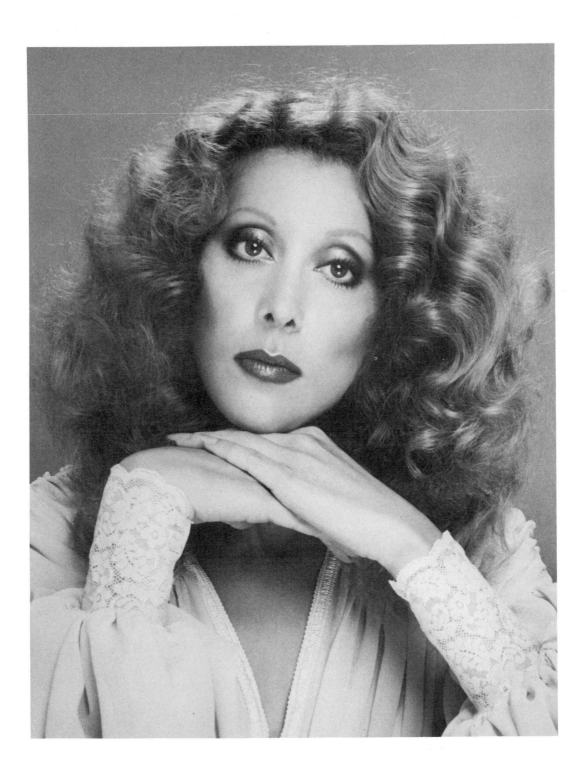

8. Rusty brown eye shadow to exaggerate the crease of the lid and to darken outer corners; lighter rusty brown shadow on lid and shimmery iridescent bronze on center of her lids for an extra glow and a smoky effect; golden tan shadow on brow bone; no inner eye liner; dark brown eye liner top and bottom.

9. Silverized and light brown eyebrow pencils applied with very short strokes in the direction in which the hairs would grow naturally.

10. Dark brown lip liner; brown lipstick; no lip gloss.

STEP 10

LIPS

Outline the lips with a lip pencil. Using a lip brush, color your lips with your chosen shade, and follow with an application of gloss.

In a recent survey conducted by a national women's magazine, 23 percent of the men questioned said they are first attracted by a woman's smile. And in the same survey, 48 percent said they preferred that women wear a natural-toned lipstick rather than none at all. Creating the look of a natural, sexy mouth is easy, especially with a lip pencil and a lip brush.

Always keep the lips protected with a conditioner or lipstick. I like to apply a lip conditioner to the lips immediately before applying lipstick. Aloe vera and vegetable oils are marvelous ingredients to look for in a conditioner. These emollients help soften and smooth even the driest lips.

Before lining the lips, it is important that the area above the upper lip is free of excess hair (I'll discuss this process later on). The object is to have a clean lip line. Also before applying lip liner, I sometimes define the crest of the upper lip with a light beige lip liner pencil (photo A). This is an optional step that you can use for evening.

Before applying color, make sure your mouth is covered with foundation and powder, a precaution that will prevent your lipstick from running and help it last longer. The foundation will also conceal the natural lip line so you can make your lips look thinner or fuller if necessary.

The shade of lip liner you buy should be as close to your natural lip color as possible. It should also be close to the shade of lipstick you'll be wearing. I find that a reddish brown shade usually meets both criteria. No one brand seems to be better than the other, so don't spend a fortune on a lip pencil. Beauty supply houses offer a wide selection of inexpensive pencils. Just be sure they're not too dry, and keep them well-sharpened.

For the most natural look, draw the line right on your own lip line (photo B). You can make small or thin lips appear larger by following the natural contours of your mouth slightly outside your natural lip line. And, conversely, you'll create the illusion of thinner lips by drawing the line just inside your

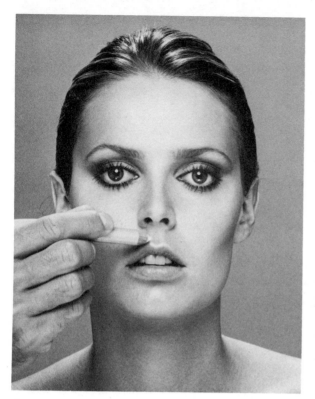

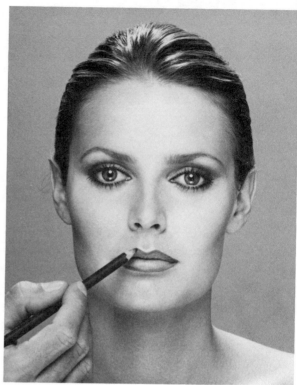

A   B

natural lip line. You can only cheat a bit—drawing a lip line too different than your own could make you look like a clown.

Britt Ekland is a perfect example of a woman with full, lush lips. In fact, it's one of her most striking features. Britt doesn't try to minimize the fullness of her lips, but she does use a pale shade of lipstick, which subdues the look.

Avoid making the bow of the upper lip too pointed. Ideally, the highest point of the curve should be directly under the center of each nostril.

Women tend to look too made up when their lipstick is either too bright or too dark. A subdued mouth always gives the impression of less makeup. Reserve a more pronounced mouth for special occasions, low light conditions, or for those times when you really want to make a fashion statement.

When selecting a lipstick color, it is not necessary to match it to your blusher or eye shadow, but do coordinate the shades. Peach-colored lipstick looks odd with plum eye shadow or rosy blusher; but pink lipstick, rose blusher, and plum shadow complement each other. On the other hand, it is disconcerting to see a woman in an orange dress wear red lipstick. Redheads should usually avoid pale pink and fuchsia lipsticks—orangish shades of red are better for them.

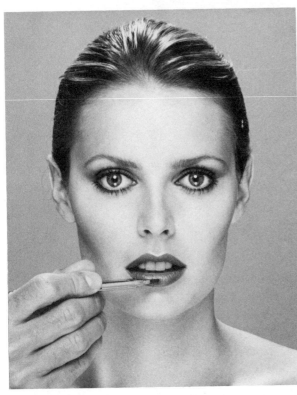

C

Step 10: Lips

Remember that bright lipsticks tend to make the mouth more prominent and that dark shades generally accentuate. A very dark red or dark brown can make full lips look fuller and thin lips look thinner.

Experiment with your lip colors. Try blending one shade of lipstick over another. If your new red lipstick is too bright, tone it down by wearing it over or under a brown or beige shade. Applying a coat of yellow lip color under lipstick will prevent it from turning purple. Also, avoid true orange shades, as they tend to make teeth look yellow.

Though I'm not a fan of frosted lipsticks, they do serve a purpose. A frosted shade, worn over a matte color, can act as a highlighter, making the lips look fuller. You can achieve the same effect by blending pure white lip color in the center of the bottom lip, making it appear fuller.

My favorite type of lip color is lipstick, and I prefer using a lip brush to apply it. The brush not only makes it easy to define the shape of the mouth, it also allows you to control the amount of color. The retractable lip brushes sold in most beauty supply stores work nicely and are never messy. Just be sure the bristles are short and firm.

Fill in your outlined lips with the lip color (photo C), extending just to the

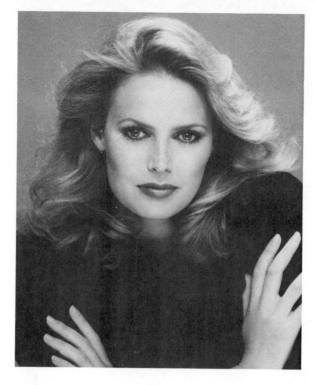

Ten steps later, our model, Lesa Weis, looks dramatically different from the way she did when we began, but she still has a fresh, natural look. For this photo, stylist Michael Macahilig set Lesa's fine, straight hair in large hot rollers, then back brushed for fullness.

outline but not over it, since the lip liner will prevent the lipstick from "bleeding." It is not necessary to blot your entire mouth by pressing the lips together over a tissue—this removes too much color. If you want to remove some lip color, gently *pat* the lips with a tissue.

Here are a few lip color tips:

- For the longest-lasting color, use your lip liner pencil to color in both lips, then blend with a fingertip.
- Coat your lipstick brush from the sides of the lipstick, in long, gentle strokes. This way your lipstick will retain its shape.
- For a non-glossy look, apply lipstick, pat gently with a tissue, apply a little translucent powder, add more lipstick, and repeat the powder, finishing with a coat of lipstick. The result is a long-lasting application with a matte finish.
- If your lipstick breaks, heat the ends over a flame until the lipstick begins to melt, then press the ends together and let it cool in the refrigerator.

Unless your lips are very dry, don't select a combination lipstick/gloss. The effect is not as natural as the translucent look of clear or tinted gloss worn over lipstick. Petroleum jelly can be substituted for lip gloss.

LYNDA CARTER

LYNDA'S NATURAL FEATURES
Wide face
High cheekbones
Round cheeks
Naturally dark lashes and brows
Very light green eyes
Tiny upturned nose that can look wide from some angles
Slightly thin upper lip

Lynda Carter is a perfect Wonder Woman, full of beauty and humor. She has a wonderful face with huge eyes, but without the proper makeup, her mouth gets lost. I created a balance by adding more fullness to her upper lip. Reddish brown lip liner extends over the center bow of the upper lip and follows slightly outside her natural lip line to the outer corners.

Lynda, a stunning actress and entertainer, is also the fashion and beauty director for Maybelline. She tests new products, helps develop color schemes, and acts as a liaison between the company and the public.

Lynda, a five-foot-nine-inch beauty, lives on a ranch and foregoes wearing makeup when she's at home. "But if I'm going to be seen, I try to look terrific. I wear makeup whenever I go anywhere. I can do a full makeup for stage in half an hour. For everyday, it takes me about ten or fifteen minutes."

Lynda confesses that it doesn't take too much discipline to keep her body in shape—she was blessed with a great figure. Of course, she admits, her active lifestyle, which includes swimming, running, playing tennis, and working out, burns extra calories. "I put on weight quickly, but I take it off just as quickly. It isn't unusual for me to put on six pounds in one night if I go on a binge, but by eating carefully the next two days, I'm back to normal. Actually, I rarely binge. I also eat very little meat, I stay away from fats and oils, and I steam all vegetables." She attributes her blemish-free skin to consistent skin care and drinking lots of water. ("I bet I drink a gallon a day.")

For her after photo, Hugh York added volume to Lynda's fine rich brown hair by using hot rollers and back brushing.

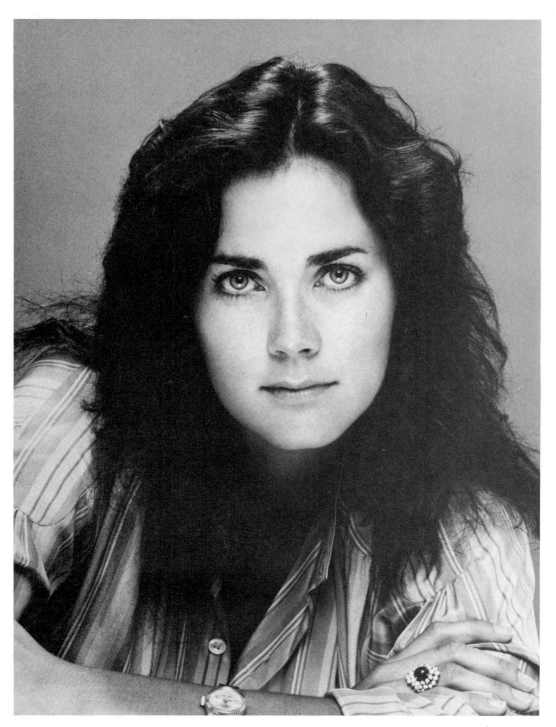

Lynda Carter

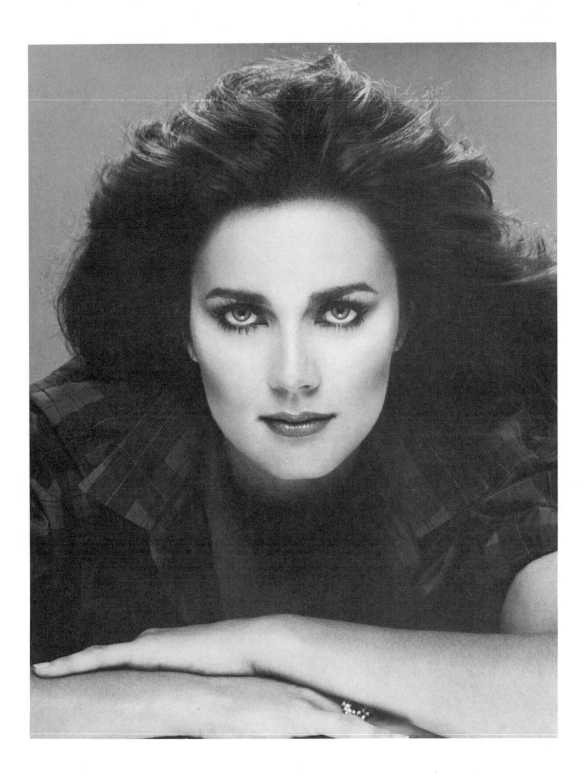

1. No blemish cover.
2. No concealer.
3. Beige liquid foundation to even her skin tone.
4. Highlighter above cheekbones angled upward toward the temples and also under the hollows of her cheeks to emphasize the jawbone and create more angles on her face.
5. Contour shadow on the temples and under the cheekbones.
6. Translucent face powder.
7. Pink blusher on cheeks, chin, and temples.
7A. Neutral brown contour shadow on the sides of her nose; highlighter from the bridge to the tip.
8. Dark, muted lavender eye shadow on the crease of the lid, extending upward and out to create a more slanted eye; pinkish lavender shadow on the center of the lid; gray shadow on the outer corners of the lid; neutral brown on the inner corners of the lid, blended carefully toward the bridge of her nose; black inner and outer eye liner on both top and bottom lids; one coat of black mascara.
9. Charcoal eyebrow pencil at the ends of her brow to lengthen them slightly.
10. Highlight pencil to define the crest of the lip; reddish brown lip liner extending over the center of her upper lip creates fullness; reddish brown lipstick; gloss.

GINGER RAABE

GINGER'S NATURAL FEATURES
Close-set, round green eyes
Full brows
High cheekbones
Cute, turned-up nose
Full, sexy lips

When Ginger Raabe wanted to dress up, this pretty homemaker and mother of two wasn't confident about her makeup. Her biggest question was about lipstick: "Should I wear it or shouldn't I? My lips are so full." I told her that her mouth was one of her nicest features, that her full lips were sexy. I also showed her how to outline them slightly inside her natural lip line to minimize the fullness. I suggested a pale, natural-looking lipstick that accents her sexy pout.

Pulling the back of her hair up off the neck draws attention to her beautiful green eyes, which I emphasized with several shades of lavender eye shadow.

Ginger's Makeup

1. No blemish cover.
2. No concealer.
3. Medium beige liquid foundation.
4. Highlighter above her cheekbones and at the inner corners of the eyes.
5. Contour shadow under her naturally high cheekbones to emphasize them.
6. Translucent face powder.
7. Soft pink blusher on her cheeks and chin and on the bridge of her nose.
8. Lavender eye shadow in the crease of the lid, blending up toward the brow; light lavender on the lid; light lavender inner liner on the bottom lids only; muted purple eye liner on the outer corners only of both top and bottom lids, smudged slightly; two coats of black mascara.
9. No eyebrow pencil.
10. Beige lip liner inside the natural lip line on both top and bottom to slightly minimize her full lips; beige lipstick; pink gloss.

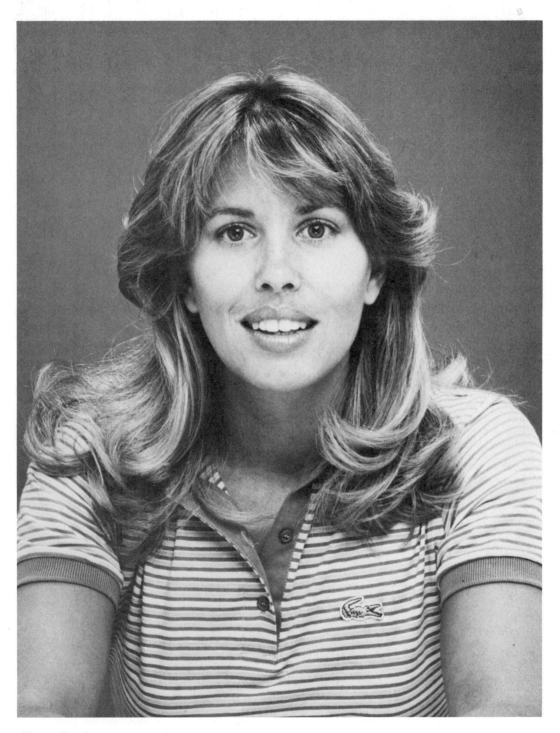

Ginger Raabe

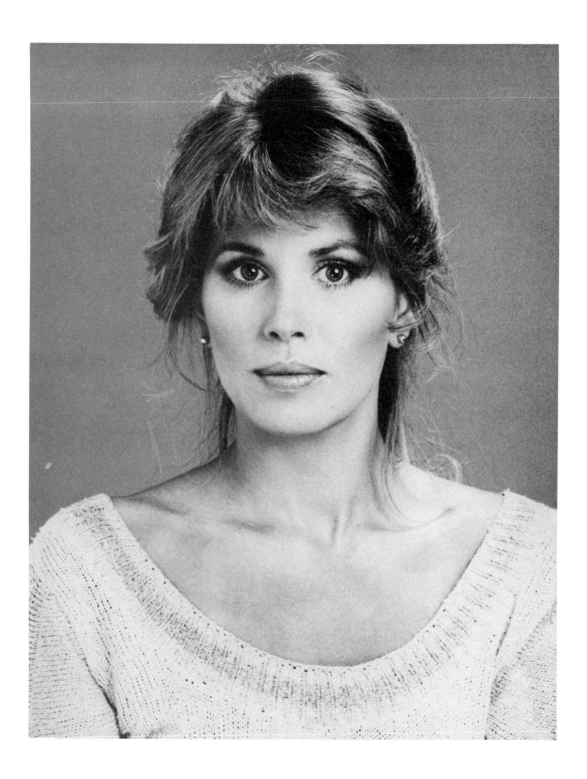

3

HAIR: THE LONG AND SHORT OF IT

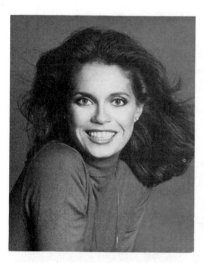
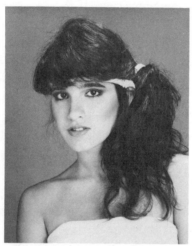
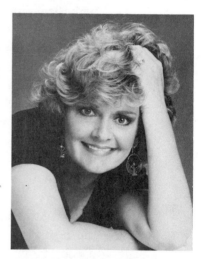
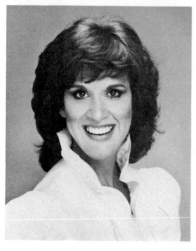
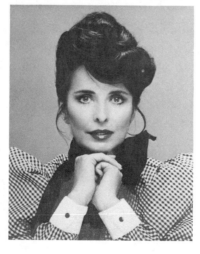
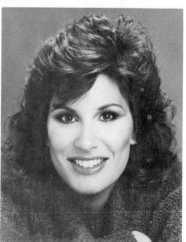

Your hairstyle can help you look casual, sophisticated, sexy, sporty, or businesslike—or give you whatever image you want. Sometimes I advise my clients to go to the best salon they can find, particularly the first time. Your hair is important; and a stylist's talent and experience can make a world of difference in your appearance.

Style: Have It Your Way

Just as you wouldn't tell a dress designer how to make a dress for you, you can't tell a hair stylist how to give you a hairstyle. That's unfair. Tell your stylist about yourself, about the way you live, about your hair and its little idiosyncracies. If he or she wants to give you bangs and you're not comfortable with them, ask for an alternative. If you like to sleep late in the morning and only allow yourself fifteen minutes to get ready, tell your stylist you need a super-easy hairdo that you won't have to fuss with every morning. A professional needs to know if you wash your hair daily, whether you can handle a blow dryer or not, if you like a versatile style that can be worn many ways, if the left side of your hair curls better than the right, and any other important bits of information only you can provide. If you've seen hairstyles that you'd like to try, take in several pictures and discuss the pros and cons of that look to give your stylist an idea of what you have in mind. Remember, above all, he or she wants to please you so you'll come back.

Don't be afraid to ask what your stylist is going to do before he or she begins. Ask how the hairdo will complement your long (or short) neck. Will the new style offset your square jawline? Can you wear bangs with your glasses? How can your hair make your eyes look bigger? Will the cut look good wet or dry?

Sometimes, limp, fine hair can be aided by perms, which can add the look of more volume, while wiry, coarse hair can be temporarily tamed with conditioners. But in all cases, a great cut minimizes problems and maximizes your natural beauty assets.

Ask your stylist to show you how to trim your own split ends and bangs to prolong the life of your initial cut. Keep in mind that a cut that requires frequent trimming is not practical on a tight budget.

The Kindest Cut

Very few people have the round, oval, square, oblong, and heart-shaped faces that beauty experts have described for so many years. And trying to match their face to one of those silly face-shape diagrams drives most women crazy. First of all, realize that there is no "perfect" shape for a face. The secret is *balance*. Trying to conform to an oval because someone says that's the best shape for a face is a never-ending battle. Be happy with the gorgeous face you've got and find a hairstyle that balances it best.

Here are a few basics to remember:

- Very short hair or hair pulled back off the face accentuates features and the actual shape of your face. A fuller hairstyle calls attention to the hair itself, helping to minimize prominent features.
- If your cheeks are full, a longer hairstyle with an angular cut can be very flattering.
- Hair that falls forward tends to diminish a full face, while a "bowl" cut can accentuate its roundness.
- If your face is long, bangs will give it a shorter look.
- Narrow faces appear fuller when the hairstyle is wide and full.
- Mature women who prefer long hair will find that upswept styles can create a more youthful look. Shorter hair is usually very flattering on older women.

As you discovered earlier, your makeup accentuates your best features. Now let your hairstyle do the same.

TO ACCENTUATE YOUR EYES:

- Frame them with long, straight bangs, which might even fringe over your brows.
- Wear waves or curls low at the temples to act as arrows pointing directly to your eyes.
- Sweep bangs to one side, which also makes your eyes the focal point of your face.

TO COMPLEMENT YOUR NOSE:

- A severe, pulled-back hairdo, perhaps a ponytail or chignon, looks fabulous if you have a wonderful profile. Wearing bangs with one of these styles will create a balanced look if your nose is prominent.
- If you don't want to call attention to your nose, avoid center parts, as they draw the eye to the center of your face.

TO MAKE THE MOST (OR THE LEAST) OF YOUR FOREHEAD:

- If you have horizontal expression lines on your forehead and these concern you, I'd suggest wearing bangs.
- A high forehead can be very dramatic and beautiful, but if you have a

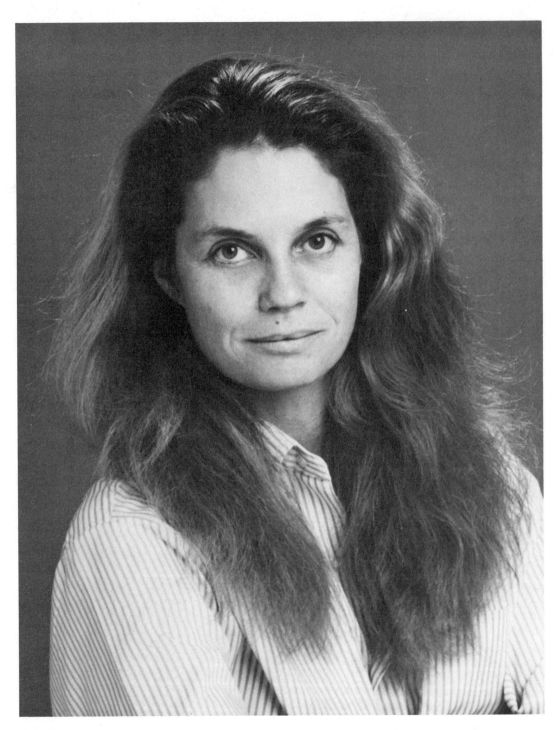

Jennifer Nairn-Smith

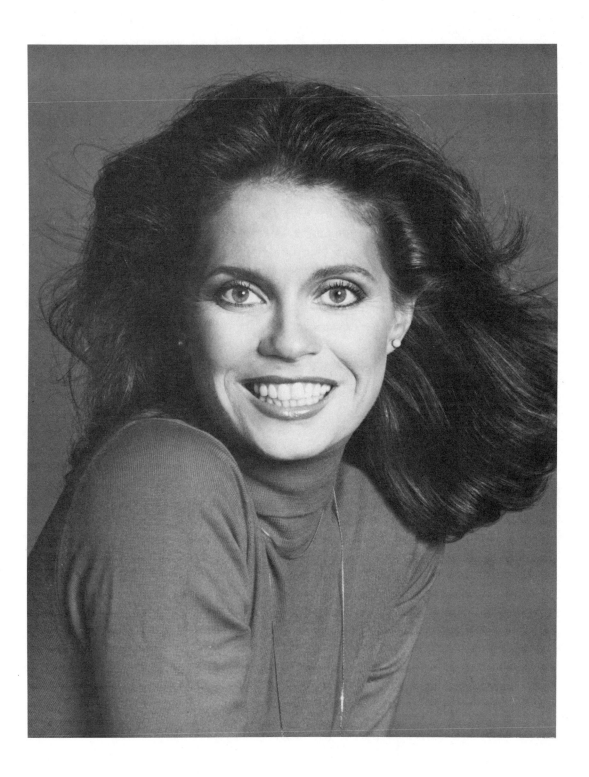

very long face, bangs work to shorten the forehead and soften the look. Also, a widow's peak can be a striking asset.

- For those with short foreheads, wear bangs that begin well above the hairline or that sweep down from high on the crown.
- Short, curly styles that frame the face but don't cover it also complement small foreheads.

TO BALANCE YOUR CHIN AND JAWLINE:

- Straight-across, squared-off bangs will accentuate a square jawline. Soft bangs that feather toward the temples will soften a strong jaw. Hair waved back and away from the face at the temples helps to balance a wide jaw, and chin-length hair will help to narrow it.
- Balance a receding chin by emphasizing the fullness on top of your head. Curls at the temples, crown, and forehead are a nice way to do that. Avoid chin-length hair; go much shorter or much longer.
- If you're troubled by one or a few too many chins, divert attention from chin level to eye level by wearing shorter hair with curls, waves, or bangs, which draw the eye upward.
- If you have a sharp, pointed, or protruding chin, create a rounded illusion by wearing chin-length hair with fullness at the chin area.

On Curls and Colors

Once you've got the right cut, then you can talk to your stylist about perms and color. Although some women are content to walk out of the salon cut and permed or cut and colored all in one sitting, others like to ease into a new look. It's up to you. But I suggest you consult a professional, especially about a perm.

I've seen more bad results from perms than I like to think about. I've seen hair that's frizzed, burned, broken, and worst of all, just plain ugly. Often professionals can tell if your hair is in the best condition for a perm. Always discuss your hair with the perm specialist, who needs to know when you last colored your hair and when you had your last perm. Most recommend a perm no more frequently than every four months.

It's rarely a good idea to color *and* perm your hair. If color is desired, wait at least ten days after a new perm.

If you decide to straighten or relax your hair, be sure your hair and scalp are in good condition and, as with a perm, never attempt a chemical treatment immediately before or after coloring.

Many women only get their hair professionally colored once and then decide that it's easier and far cheaper to do it at home. But with counseling from a professional color expert, you'll know which is the best product for your hair and which shade or shades to use. Under the proper guidance, changing your hair color doesn't have to be a traumatic experience. You can brighten your face, bring out skin tones you never knew you had, even make your clothing look better. Your skin tone and those many flecks of color in your eyes help dictate which color works best for you. With some of the new hair coloring products, you can even add body and shine to your hair.

For example, actress/dancer Jennifer Nairn-Smith, perhaps best known for her role in the film *All That Jazz,* had her hair lightened for her role in the film *The Best Little Whorehouse in Texas.* The process, however, left her hair unevenly colored, dry, and damaged. To get her hair back to a healthy and better-looking state, I suggested she have it cut to remove the damaged ends, conditioned, and darkened to its original rich, dark brown.

Although many women look magnificent with gray hair, there's no denying that it can make them look older. If you are gray and want to experiment with another color, try on some wigs first and then decide. You're safest if you stick to your original color, lightening by only one or two shades.

A colorist can "weave" or streak your hair with various tones of a lighter shade. The effect of this technique is extremely natural-looking and is the most subtle way to gradually lighten the hair or mask the gray. Since natural hair color is a combination of many shades, this method not only can look the most natural, but as the roots grow out, they aren't as obvious, so you don't have to color as often.

BEVERLY SASSOON

The curly-topped Beverly Sassoon you see in her dripping wet before shot actually has straight, dark brown hair with auburn undertones that has been permed and cut into an easy wash-and-wear style. If she lets it dry naturally, she has a soft "Grecian boy" look. For glamorous occasions, hair stylist Eric Root oils it with Tenax sculpturing lotion and sweeps it to one side, creating partial bangs that highlight her huge green eyes.

As a constantly on-the-go businesswoman, author, TV personality, and mother of four, Beverly has honed her beauty regimen to fit her tight schedule. "I love my hair short," she says. "It's easy wet or dry, and when I want it extra fluffy, all I have to do is scrunch it with my fingers."

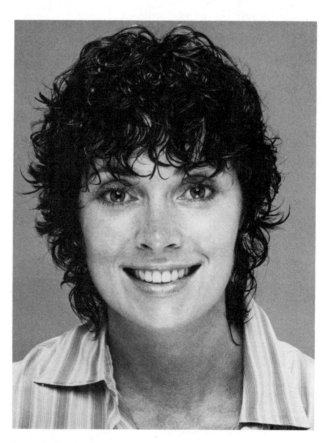

Beverly Sassoon

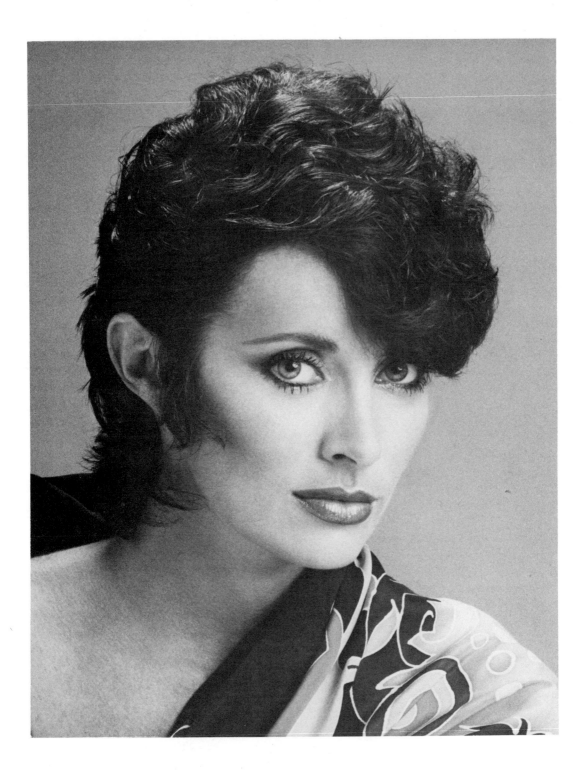

MARGARET O'BRIEN

Margaret O'Brien hasn't cut her gorgeous naturally brown hair in over eight years. Thick and straight, it falls six inches below her waist. Margaret says she's had advice from people who have suggested everything from dyeing it blond to cutting it just below her ears. "But," she says, "my hair looks best this way, because it feels right on me. I love my hair. My husband does, too." Margaret washes her hair every day using a variety of shampoos and cream rinses. She lets it dry naturally, brushing with a natural bristle brush.

Hairdresser Hugh York marveled that Margaret's hair didn't have a single

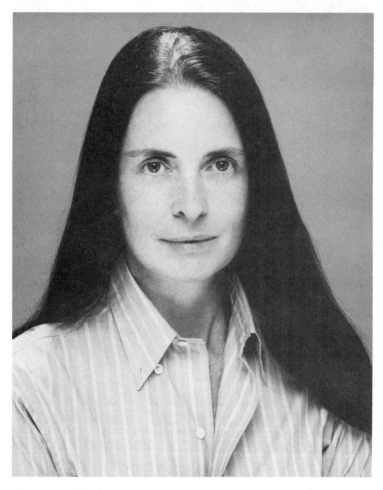

Margaret O'Brien

split end and credited that to her excellent hair care. To demonstrate how versatile long hair can be, Hugh first simply brushed her hair back, eliminating any part. Then, for a change, he styled it in a French twist, with soft fullness around her face.

A former child star, soft-spoken Margaret has retained her unaffected ingenue quality. She recalls never thinking she was pretty as a child, having always been cast as the plain little orphan. "I was always very skinny, and I think I got into the movies because I looked like I'd been through the war."

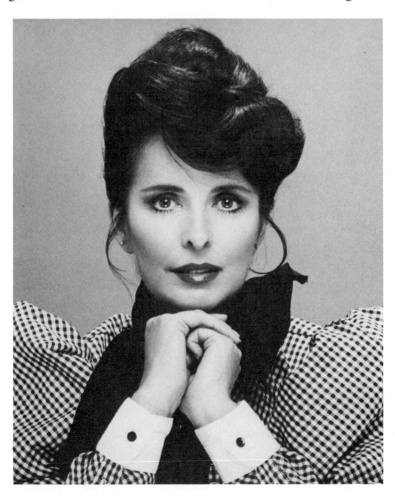

JOYCE VAN PATTEN

Joyce Van Patten makes a point of having regular cuts. "I have thick, heavy hair," Joyce notes. "My hair stylist, William Escalera, cuts and shapes my hair at least every three months and weaves in golden highlights twice a year, even though I'm naturally a blond. At home I use Redken and Nexus shampoos, alternating at every shampoo. I always give myself hot cap treatments at home, too, with Wella Kolestral and Clairol products."

To create fullness at the sides and crown to complement the shape of Joyce's face, hair stylist George Bowers used three hot rollers on top and two

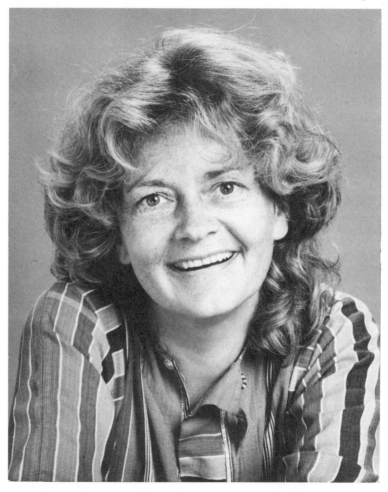

Joyce Van Patten

on each side. The secret was in the brushing. He asked her to bend over and then brushed her hair all forward from the nape of the neck. When she stood up and flicked her hair back, George simply smoothed the top a bit with his fingers.

Joyce's easy, casual hairstyle reflects her whole attitude about beauty and fashion. "Beauty is finding what you're supposed to look like and not trying to look like other people."

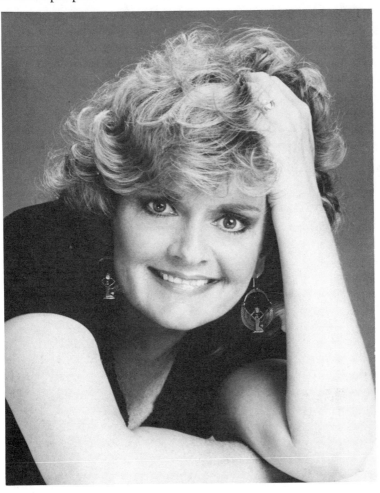

MARLENE HAMERLING

Marlene Hamerling is a free-lance copywriter in the high-energy advertising world. "I'm not a swinging single, that's for sure, but I'm always ready to look pretty," she told me.

Marlene felt that her hairstyle looked plain so hair stylist Barron gave her naturally wavy hair a bi-level cut, shorter in front than in back. With the length in back, Marlene still has the versatility of longer hair. Barron highlighted her dark hair with subtle shades of light blond and golden blond, a technique he calls "high lights and low lights." Now she can straighten her hair by using hot rollers or a blow dryer, or let her curls dry naturally after using a sculpturing lotion. After her makeover, she was beaming and tried to explain how she felt: "It's both amazing and gratifying to see yourself transformed and perfected that way. I feel beautiful, and that pervades everything else I do."

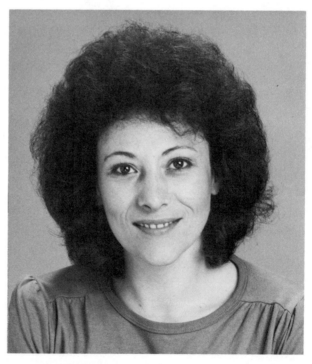

Marlene Hamerling

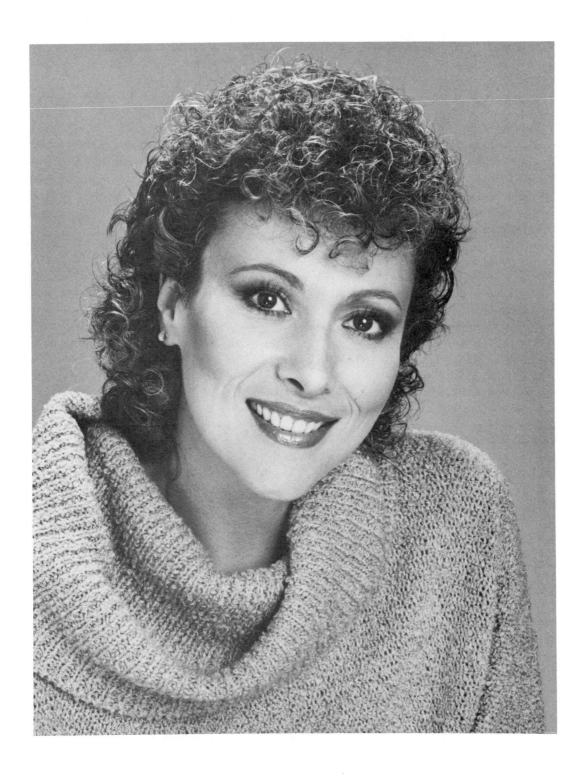

JENILEE HARRISON

Jenilee Harrison always straightened her hair for her role as Cindy Snow on TV's "Three's Company." As an actress, she needs a hairstyle that's versatile—a cut that can take her from the look of the all-American girl next door to that of the sultry sexpot. With a cut that takes advantage of her natural curl, she has the option of straightening her hair with a blow drier and then brushing, or scrunching it with her fingers into a mass of tousled curls.

To bring out the natural curl in Jenilee's hair, stylist Barron gave her a long shag cut that frames her face. Blond highlights accent her own naturally blond hair. To achieve the soft, curly style in her after photo, Jenilee used her fingers to add fullness to her hair while she let it dry naturally.

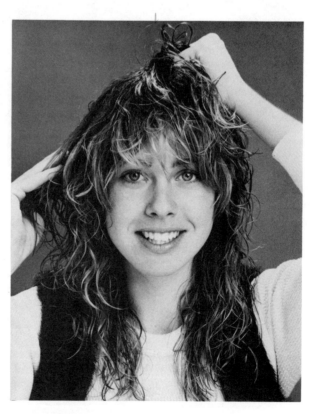

Jenilee Harrison

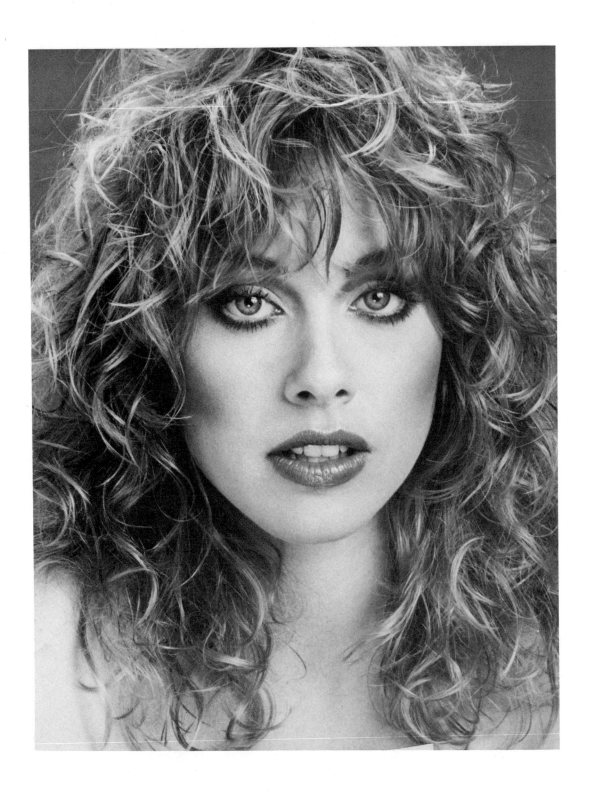

RUTH BUZZI

"Since I make most of my money by looking my worst when playing various characters, I take a great pride in how I look as Ruth Buzzi," admits the well-loved character actress/comedienne. "I have a very strange face, so I have to make the most of it."

For Ruth, looking her best is dependent on her hairstyle. "Because of this very long face of mine, I know that my hair has to be very full and especially wide at the sides. Though I wish I could wear it short, I can't—chin length is best on me." Since chin-length hair is one of the hardest cuts to handle, Ruth keeps her hair trimmed regularly. To make sure her profile looks as good as the front view, she uses a hand mirror to check her hair from all views. "If the back of my hair gets flat, my profile is awful."

Hair stylist Hugh York increased the fullness of Ruth's thick hair by using a small round brush and a blow dryer. Brushing the sides back and up also helps add width to her narrow face. Although the overall look of her cut is chin-

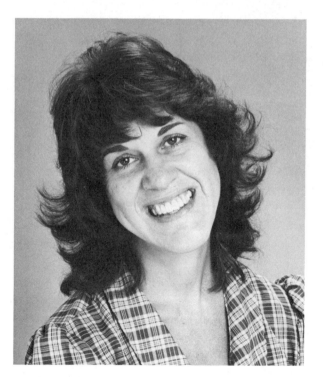

Ruth Buzzi

length, only the hair in back is actually that long. The front is short, wispy, and easy to manage.

"I color my hair myself—it's naturally a mousey brown. I mix equal parts of Miss Clairol's Sunlit Brown Number 35 and Sun Blond Brown Number 25G and leave the concoction on for twenty minutes. It gives my hair reddish highlights and actually makes it feel softer."

Ruth became a familiar face as the beloved Gladys Ormsby on the old "Laugh-In" show. She developed the character by watching real people on the street. "You'd be amazed at how many women have terrible posture and take no care with the way they dress. I would love every woman to get into Gladys garb and walk hunched over for about an hour. Then let them dress up, put on some makeup, and stand up tall. It's an easy way to go from negative to positive. It not only makes you feel like a milion bucks, it makes you feel very lucky."

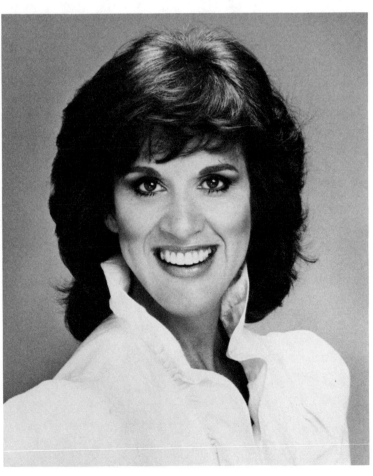

NANCY MCKEON

Nancy McKeon, at seventeen, likes a natural look. She doesn't wear a trace of makeup in her tomboy role as Jo on "The Facts of Life" and only wears a bit of it offstage. When I told her that pulling her shiny, healthy hair back off her face accentuates the roundness, she immediately pulled out the rubber band and let her fabulous dark hair tumble over her shoulders. I suggested she keep the bangs to accentuate her almond-shaped brown eyes.

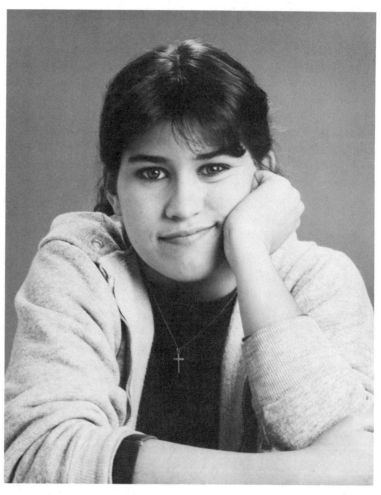

Nancy McKeon

Nancy's hair is so healthy that Jimmy Encao simply layer-cut her hair for movement and versatility. For her after photo, Nancy bent over from the waist and brushed all of her hair forward, then stood erect and smoothed it. It was a simple but significant change.

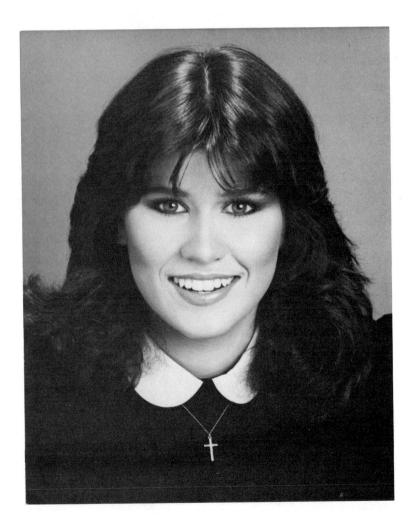

LORETTA GREENBERG

Loretta Greenberg, a secretary for a major entertainment agency, frequently sees celebrities with and without makeup, so she knows that proper makeup can work wonders. She came to see me because she wanted to see just how glamorous she could look.

I told Loretta that lightening her hair and eyebrows would make a big difference in her appearance.

Colorist Florent added highlights to Loretta's hair, "weaving" it with various shades of blond. Then stylist Barron layered her hair, leaving it at the length she loves but adding fullness at the top. Hot rollers create the soft curls Loretta wears in her after photo, but for an everyday look, she wears it soft and carefree.

We lightened her brows two shades and tweezed them, leaving more space between the brows.

Apprehensive before we started, she was delighted with the results. "It's unbelievable. The only way I know it's me is because I was there!"

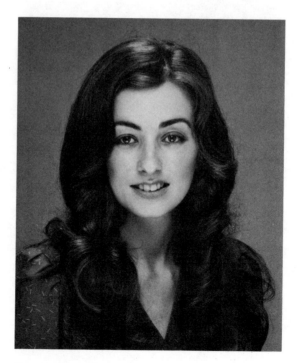

Loretta Greenberg

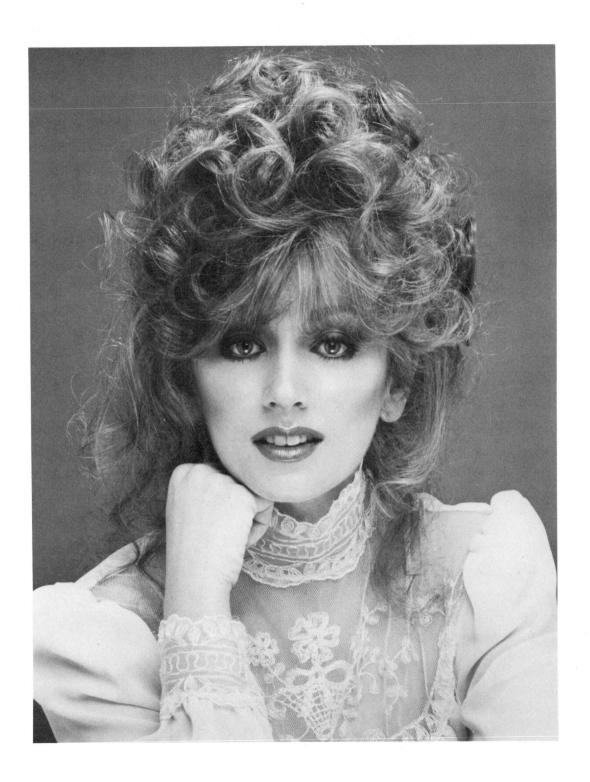

EILEEN FULTON

Eileen Fulton, who plays Lisa on "As the World Turns," is a soft-spoken southerner with a delightful manner.

When Eileen came in for her photo session, she had pinned up the back of her very fine strawberry blond hair in a style that made her high forehead look higher and her chin too long for the rest of her face. I suggested she take advantage of the length of her hair to balance her forehead and chin. Hair stylist Ramsey set her hair on large rollers, back brushed it for extra volume, smoothed it slightly, and finished with a light mist of hair spray. The width at the temples now draws attention to her eyes, while the length gives her a well-proportioned, sophisticated look.

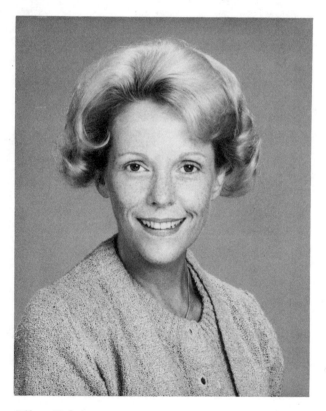

Eileen Fulton

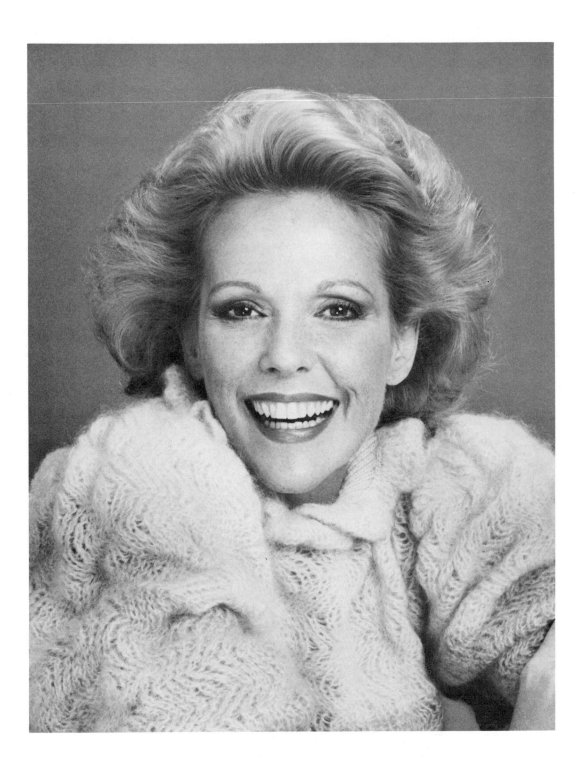

JUDY NORTON-TAYLOR

After ten years on "The Waltons," Judy Norton-Taylor wants more than just a sweet, girl-next-door look. "I've always been very critical of my appearance on the screen, but now I like my looks better than I did when I was younger. I'm confident enough now to want to try playing a strong sexy type," says Judy, who has the kind of gorgeous, thick hair that can look like a sensuous, wild mane if she's in a femme fatale mood. Because her face is broad,

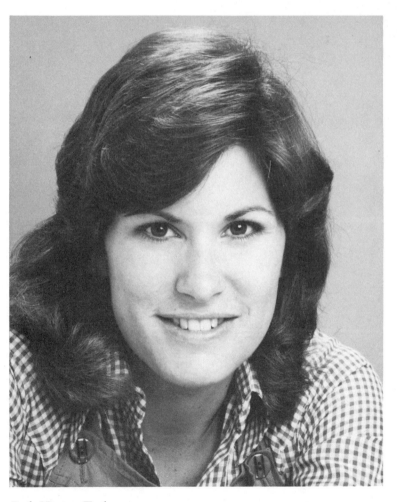

Judy Norton-Taylor

she needs a full style to balance her look. For her after photo, hair stylist John Villanueva blow dried Judy's hair, using only his fingers to comb through it. To add body to her very straight hair, he used a curling iron at the roots and about halfway down the shaft of the hair, avoiding the ends. This creates the loose, free look Judy loves.

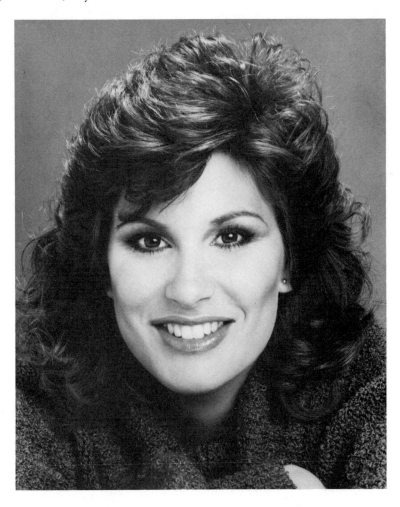

DANIELLE BRISEBOIS

After years as Archie's little niece on "Archie Bunker's Place," pretty Danielle Brisebois was ready to try something new with her thick dark brown hair. Though she likes her hair down, she says she wishes she could wear wispier bangs. Since she swims regularly and dances every day to keep in shape, stylist John Villanueva gave her an exercise-proof hairdo with those wispy bangs that she loves.

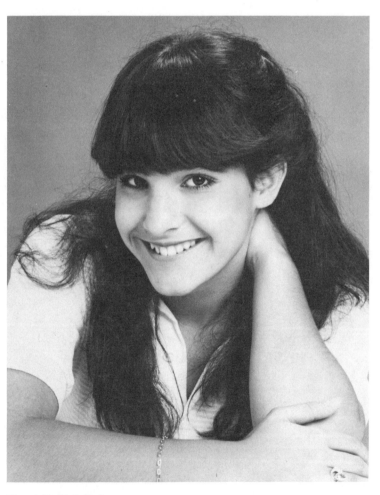

Danielle Brisebois

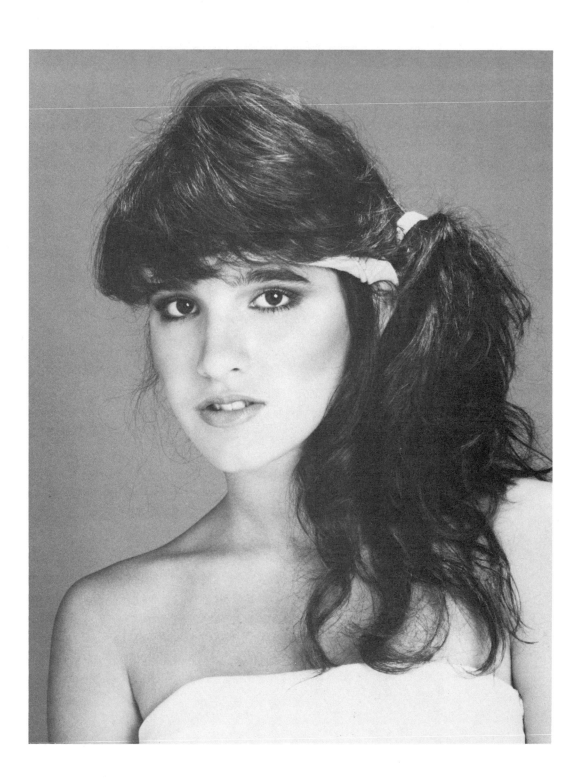

FAY DEWITT

As an actress, singer, comedienne, and mother, Fay DeWitt needs a versatile hairdo that can wear as many hats as she does. Interested in changing her naturally curly red hair and anxious for makeup advice, she came to my studio ready for a makeover. After we took her before photo, I suggested we wait about three weeks to let her hair get a bit longer and then have it professionally straightened before we shot her after photo. When she returned, we created a hairstyle that looks softer, more feminine, and youthful. This new hairdo works perfectly for her because it can look both casual or sophisticated.

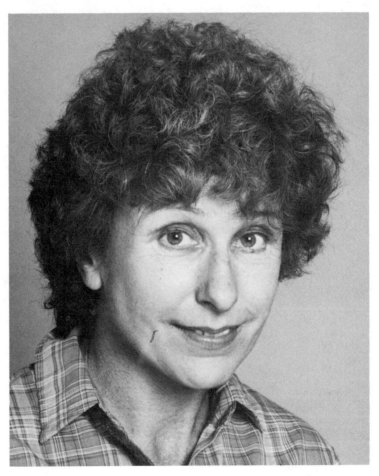

Fay DeWitt

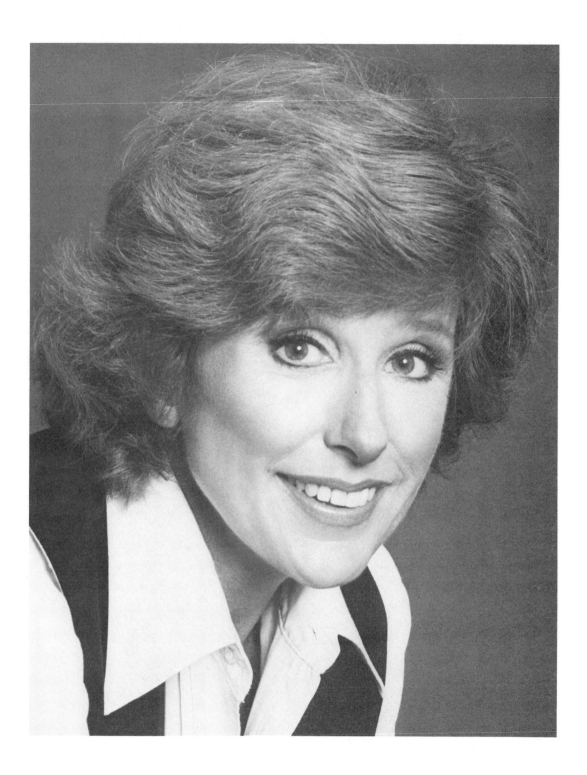

DEBORAH SHELTON

Former Miss USA Deborah Shelton has one of those gorgeous faces that needs very little done to improve it. As you can see from her before photo, she is such a natural beauty that she appears to be wearing makeup, but I can assure you she isn't. When hair stylist Michelle Lavee fixed Deborah's thick, shiny straight hair into a slick chignon, every feature was accentuated—you noticed her face and nothing else. Women whose hair is not as long as Deborah's can wear a pinned-on chignon, matched to their own hair color, and achieve equally striking results.

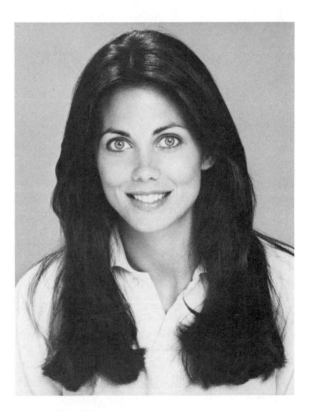

Deborah Shelton

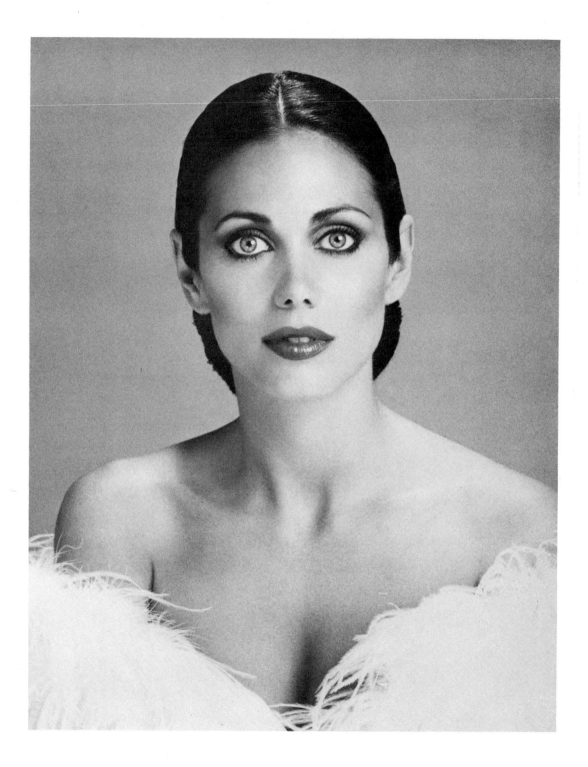

4

BEAUTY: INSIDE, OUTSIDE, HEAD TO TOE

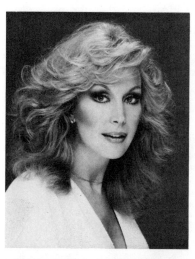
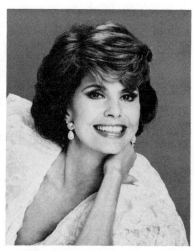
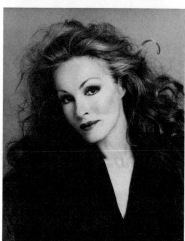
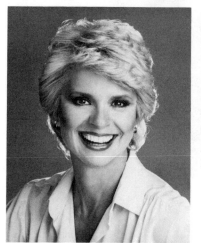
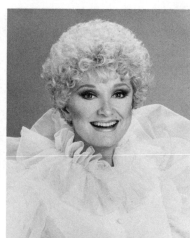
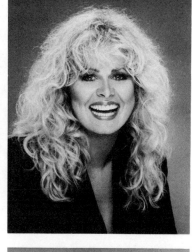

*R*ight now, go look in a full-length mirror. If you have completed your makeup and hair makeover, ask yourself, does your image from the neck down complement your new neck-up look? Be honest. Do your clothes enhance your figure? Do they fit properly? Are the colors flattering? Does your silhouette look smooth, or is it broken by a bulge here, a wrinkle there?

Does your posture express self-confidence and vitality, or do you look slouchy, tired, and ready to quit? Does the overall picture connote happiness and receptivity? Or are you blocking those feelings and closing yourself off from the rest of the world?

When superstar-maker Jay Bernstein looks for star quality, he seeks out the type of person who is so in touch with her own image that she projects it in her appearance, in her attitude, and in the way she communicates with others. Donna Dixon, whom he discovered and who is best-known for her role as Sonny on TV's "Bosom Buddies," is a perfect example of just such a star.

Think about your interaction with others. When was the last time you smiled at a stranger before he or she smiled at you? How would someone else describe you? The answers to these questions will give you some important insights about yourself. And if you're not completely satisfied with your own

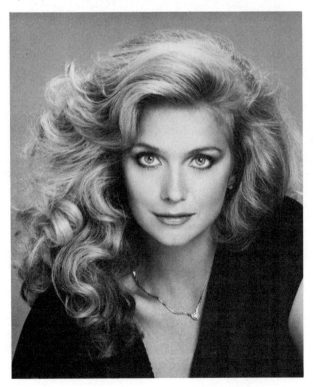

Donna Dixon
(Hairstyle by Ramsey)

responses, consider making some changes in the all-important area of self-confidence.

Dressing for Impact

Obviously, your wardrobe has a lot to say about you. The impact of clothing is easy to illustrate with photographs. I'll show you how a change of blouse or shoes or even a handbag can change the look of your figure. Knowing that you look your best from head to toe is one of the first steps in instilling self-confidence.

Dr. Joyce Brothers explains how her clothes affect her: "If I have a run in my stocking or a stain on my blouse—even the kind nobody else notices—or if I'm overdressed or underdressed, it robs attention from what I'm doing and shifts my focus to how I look. Once I put myself together in the morning and I feel I'm dressed properly, I never want to think about the way I look. I want to concentrate on what I'm doing. My clothes should be like the watch on my wrist: It's there all day doing its job, but I never have to think about it."

You know you're dressed properly when you look in that full-length mirror and the first thing you see is your face. Not a hem that's falling, a print that's too overpowering, a neckline that's too low or too high, or a bulge where your bra strap is cutting into your shoulder. Your clothes can be interesting and indicate something about your personality, but they shouldn't say anything more forcefully than you can with your face alone.

Proper Fit

First, stop thinking about numbers. What difference does it make if you buy a size 8, 10, or 12 if the clothing fits? Every manufacturer will tell you that the same size can vary as much as two inches from company to company. So even if you have to buy size 14 Calvin Klein jeans, size 10 shorts at Penney's, and size 12 slacks by Liz Claiborne, do you really care what size they are as long as they fit properly? Let the mirror tell you what fits. Tight clothes that gap and wrinkle magnify your figure flaws, making you look heavier than you really are.

Clothes that are too big can be just as disastrous. When your clothes fit properly, they look and feel new. A tailor can do wonders just by adjusting a shoulder, lifting a hem, taking in a seam, letting one out, or by controlling the fullness in a sleeve or skirt. The adjustments may be major or minor, but the results can change the entire look of your garment—and your image.

Mentioning the Unmentionables

Most fine department stores still have specialists who will help you find exactly the right size and style foundation to make your figure look its best and to make your clothes fit properly. There are bras to minimize the large bust as well as padded styles to maximize smaller bosoms. Sometimes a change of bra is all that's necessary to alleviate gapping spaces between buttons or the stress wrinkles that occur when a garment is just a smidge too tight. Body stockings, those sheer, all-in-one garments, can help you look ten pounds thinner and create one clean line from bustline to hem.

Planning a Wardrobe

You've heard it said many times before: You don't need a lot of expensive clothes to have a wonderful wardrobe. Like anything else that's important to you, it takes thought, time, and careful planning. If you're like Lynda Carter and hate to shop, take advantage of the personal shoppers who are employed by most department stores. Make an appointment to discuss your specific needs. Bring an inventory of your wardrobe, listing your favorite pieces, and let the shopper help you add a few that will work with your old favorites to create more versatility in your closet.

I talked to some of the most creative names in the world of fashion to hear how they suggest putting together a versatile, practical, and fabulous wardrobe.

Bob Mackie, whose glamorous designs have graced the bodies of many of Hollywood's most beautiful women, takes a surprisingly ultra-classic, tailored approach to building a workable wardrobe. In fact, he told me that women spend too much money on special-occasion clothes and not enough on their everyday things. He suggests that women invest in a few basic articles of clothing using one color scheme. Here, for instance, is Bob Mackie's complete go-anywhere wardrobe:

- a navy blue skirted suit
- a gray skirt
- a pair of gray slacks
- a red blazer
- a navy or gray cardigan sweater
- a tailored red blouse
- a tailored white blouse
- a gray V-neck pullover
- a navy turtleneck

Mackie says that by combining any two or three of these pieces, you can rest assured that you're well-dressed for most occasions. The same plan can work in another color scheme, such as ivory, black, and light blue; or beige, rust, and brown.

Designer Geoffrey Beene told me that comfort should be the prime consideration when selecting a wardrobe. "If a person is not comfortable in his or her clothes, the clothes are not serving the purpose for which they were designed. For instance, I would much rather see a woman wearing soft pajama pants in the evening than a strapless gown in which she does not feel free to move."

The color scheme of a wardrobe is of primary importance to designer Liz Claiborne, who dresses more working women in America than any other single designer. "Think about colors so that everything in your closet can work with everything else. Don't buy a blue item this week and an orange one the next. Plan purchases carefully. Investment pieces such as jackets should be in neutral colors that go with many different items in the wardrobe. Navy blue is a good choice, but so is an interesting tweed that picks up many of the colors you enjoy wearing. Naturally, the colors you select as the foundation of your wardrobe should be colors that look good on *you,* not shades you have chosen because they are 'in' at the moment."

Image consultant Alayne Harris has spent years studying the effects of color on the human form and psyche. "Mustard yellow is the most universally disliked color as well as the least flattering color to the largest number of people," she says. "Next to mustard, the most aggravating color seems to be orange. This information can be put to good use. You see orange decor in many fast food chains. Since orange is so psychologically irritating, people want to leave the restaurant quickly. That means frequent turnover. In the restaurant industry, they call it 'hungry orange.' The colors we wear have the same kind of psychological impact, and we can use color to create subtle influences."

Alayne goes on to explain that beige, tan, camel, buff, soft blue, and yellow are called the likability colors, with yellow rating highest. Black and dark colors have a cold value, which tend to keep people at a distance. Interpreting this information, it would seem clear that yellow, soft blue, or neutrals might be the best colors to wear on a job interview and that black or navy would work for a power image.

What's Your Style?

The women I photograph have their own fashion styles: Linda Gray, who plays Sue Ellen Ewing on TV's "Dallas," explains that she dresses to suit her mood, not necessarily to keep up with fashion. "I keep up with what I love. I like to mix and match so nobody can predict what I'll be wearing. I think that's style. One day I may feel like a gypsy and I may wear a long skirt and an ethnic blouse, and the next day I may feel conservative and put on a suit."

Betty White is another woman who doesn't follow fashion trends. "I feel best in tailored blouses with soft scarves and wear blouses and skirts most of the time," she explains. "I will wear pants occasionally, but I don't feel comfortable in jeans. I don't wear furs because I love animals and I don't believe in taking their skins. I enjoy soft fabrics and soft colors, especially blue, green and peach."

When Carol Burnett talks about clothes, she mentions Adolfo and Missoni as two of her favorite designers. "But I don't buy many clothes. I buy things that I truly like. If I get tired of them or they go out of style, I put them in the closet for a while. I'm most comfortable in jeans and a soft cotton top."

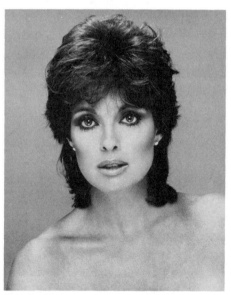

Linda Gray (*Hairstyle by Jose Eber*)

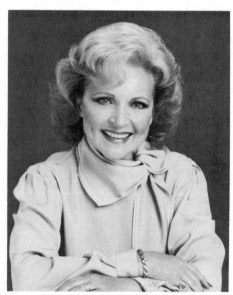

Betty White

Beautiful Cheryl Ladd opts for a high-fashion look and loves the clean, geometric lines of clothes by Italian designer Giorgio Armani and New York's avant-garde Norma Kamali. "I'm probably most comfortable in jeans," Cheryl admitted, "but after making a film about Kentucky coal miners, in which I had to wear dungarees all the time, I am now very partial to dresses."

Cyd Charisse, who for years has been known as one of the most fashionable women in Hollywood, tells me she prefers a soft, feminine look and loves silks, romantic ruffles, delicate colors, and subtle prints.

Eileen Ford, head of one of the world's largest modeling agencies, makes an interesting point when she talks about fashion. "You don't have to buy high-priced designer clothes to look fashionable. You can make your own clothes—Butterick, Simplicity, McCall, and Vogue all offer designer patterns. There are discount stores all over the country that sell designer clothes at reduced prices. J. C. Penney and Spiegel are projecting a strong fashion image these days by presenting designer clothes at realistic prices. You have to be a creative shopper—one who doesn't just look for high price tags to connote good value."

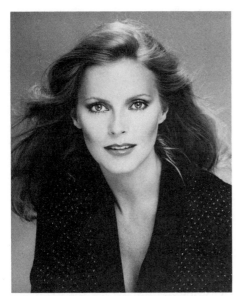

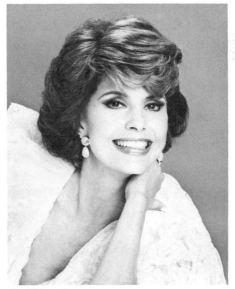

Cheryl Ladd (*Hairstyle by Ramsey*)   **Cyd Charisse** (*Hairstyle by Richard Bradshaw*)

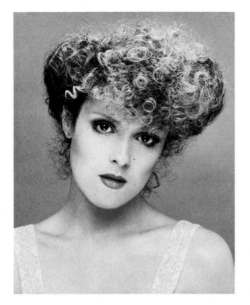

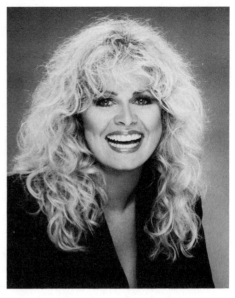

Bernadette Peters
(Hairstyle by Allen Edwards)

Sally Struthers *(Hairstyle by Hakudo Isoda)*

Great Looks for Short Women

Most people don't believe it when Bernadette Peters tells them she's only five-foot-two. "I wear form-fitting clothes because they make me look taller. I had to learn how to dress for my height and how to reject some beautiful things that were made for six-foot-tall models."

Similarly petite, Sally Struthers understands her figure so well that she knows exactly what to wear. "I'm short—five feet one and a half inches—I have a round face and a large bust, so I have to be careful how I dress. I avoid turtlenecks or anything with a round neckline. Usually the best neckline for me is a V-neck. Recently I found that by tucking shoulder pads under my bra straps, I create more width at the shoulders and more angles, which help balance my bustline—I appear slimmer. I also try to dress monochromatically, which makes me look taller. That helps, since my weight often fluctuates fifteen pounds up or down. That looks like thirty pounds on me because I'm so short."

For years, the fashion industry overlooked over half of the world's women—the half under five feet four inches. Evey petite woman who comes into my studio eventually complains that clothes were made for the five-foot-eight-and-over mannequins with birch-tree figures. Good conscience and/or good sense finally caught up with the fashion industry a few years ago, and many designers have entered the world of fashions for petites. Many of the same clothes that look fabulous on taller women are now available in smaller sizes. So it's no longer necessary for short women to dress in styles that don't express sophisticated attitudes. By careful shopping and by following some simple guidelines, you can dress to complement your size.

LONG ILLUSIONS

- Avoid wearing dresses, suits, or pants in bulky fabrics. This is *not* to say that you must avoid wearing thick, fuzzy sweaters, textured skirts, or a luxurious quilted jacket. Just make sure that you wear slim pants with your hand-knit sweaters, a sleek silk shirt with that heavy skirt, or a narrow evening skirt or pants with your quilted jacket.

- Wear similar shades from waist to toe, but don't feel you must restrict yourself to wearing one color from head to toe. Perhaps your chosen outfit is a red sweater and gray flannel skirt. In this case, instead of wearing the usual natural-toned hosiery, opt for pearl gray sheer or opaque stockings and charcoal leather pumps. Or charcoal gray rib-knit stockings and black oxfords. If you choose to wear slacks, wear a neutral boot or shoe that blends with the color of your pants. Since the length of most jackets falls below your waist, they should blend with the shade of your skirt or slacks. No need to match, just blend. If your jacket is shorter than waist length, it can contrast with what you're wearing. Here, again, it's okay for the short jacket to match or blend with the bottom, but you needn't feel compelled to wear all one color.

- Make sure that what you wear is in proportion to your size. Generally avoid large handbags, no clunky shoes, super-high heels, enormous floral prints, huge hats, very wide skirts, below-the-hip jackets, six-inch-wide belts, and extreme collars. You can wear short skirts, long skirts, or knee-length skirts; you can wear sweaters, blouses, jackets, and tops with high necks, low necks, V-necks, square necks, round necks, even turtlenecks. Just avoid extremes.

- Don't try to be something you're not. You're not tall. Concentrate on being yourself. People respond to your personality and achievements, not to your height. Height didn't get in the way of some of the world's most stunning women, including petite Barbara Eden, whose height—five foot two—surprises most people. Nancy Reagan has to be one of the most elegant women in the world, and she certainly isn't tall.

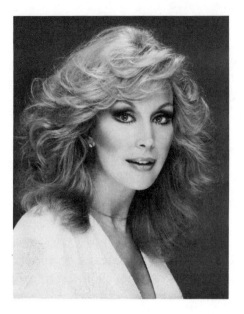

Barbara Eden (*Hairstyle by Gayle Rowell*)

Dressing Tall

Vertical lines make you look taller. Also keep in mind that horizontal stripes will give you a wider, slightly shorter look. All-one-color outfits create a long line; different colors at top and bottom break up the body. If you want to play up the fact that you're tall, take the one-color, vertical approach—long, lean tunics or equally lean trousers, or very narrow, long skirts with cardigans, stockings that blend with your skirts. If you want to appear less tall, take a subtly horizontal approach—wide shoulders, broad belts, full skirts, boxy jackets.

Big and Beautiful

Carole Shaw, editor of *Big Beautiful Woman* magazine, a fashion journal geared for the large woman, says there's no reason a woman can't be beautiful and dressed well at any size. In her magazine, Carole works with large-size models, most of whom wear size 18 or larger and dresses them in clothes that break all the rules of camouflage. "Why hide?" she asks. She puts belts on her models, she tucks in their blouses, she lets them wear horizontal stripes, she advocates vivid colors, and she tells them to throw away their polyester pull-on pants. Instead of trying to hide their bodies, Carole liberates them and shows women who have been ashamed of their extra pounds exactly how lovely they can look. This is my approach to every woman who walks into my studio—"Be as beautiful as you can be, starting right now!"

Body Balancing

Fashion coordinator Andrea Sells worked with me coordinating the fashion makeovers in this section.

Most women are troubled by spot problems, such as large hips, a thick waist, or a large bust. By minimizing the problem areas and highlighting your assets, your figure can look its best. Here are some of the problems you may have and the solutions that can counterbalance them.

ROUND FACE: If your face looks too round, a V-neckline is usually the most flattering. Wearing button-front shirts and leaving the top one or two buttons open will also create a longer illusion. Avoid turtlenecks or extremely high collars.

LONG FACE: Scoop necklines and high turtlenecks both complement a long face. So does a man-tailored shirt, buttoned high and worn with a soft bow at the neck. Long faces also look terrific in full cowl necklines that drape softly in front at the chin line. Avoid V- and U-necklines as well as long, pointed collars, which will tend to elongate your face.

LONG NECK: You have the advantage of being able to wear almost any neckline. Low backs look especially graceful on you, since they emphasize the long line created from the nape of your neck to the small of your back. If you want to shorten the look of your neck, wear high turtlenecks, ruffled Victorian collars, or any style with lots of details at the neckline.

SHORT NECK: Expose as much as possible of your neck; opt for V-necks, U-necks, or scooped necklines instead. If you like the look of soft, Victorian styles, find those that do not band the throat, with narrow ruffles falling as low as possible on the neckline. Avoid short necklaces that seem to break up the line of the neck.

NARROW SHOULDERS: You can wear dolman sleeves. raglan sleeves, and any of the exaggerated padded-shoulder styles. If you keep the line below your waist extremely narrow (i.e., jeans, straight skirts, shorts), you can wear halter tops, but avoid full-skirted, halter-top dresses, as they accentuate your narrow shoulder line.

BROAD SHOULDERS: Good fit is extremely important. Take the time to have a tailor check the fit of your investment pieces—your blazers, good dresses, and special blouses. A tailor can move the shoulder line slightly to create a narrower look. Anything too big will make your shoulders look wider. Avoid broad shoulder pads. Avoid horizontal yokes and dolman sleeves. If you love puffed sleeve looks, have a tailor adjust the fullness so you don't look like a football player.

ROUND SHOULDERS: Anything that defines your shoulders, such as pert puffed sleeves, shoulder pads, crisp fabrics, and large, square collars will straighten out your shoulder line. Avoid raglan and dolman sleeves and halter necklines—these accentuate a round line.

LARGE BUST: A V-neck is again one of the most flattering. Select soft fluid fabrics in solid colors or subtle prints. Wear earrings to draw the eye up toward your face. Stay away from horizontal seaming on blouses, since that calls attention to the bustline and creates a wider illusion. Avoid chest pockets, large ruffles, and high, round necklines. If you want to wear a dolman sleeve and your shoulders slope, try using soft shoulder pads, as Sally Struthers suggested.

SMALL BUST: Go after a curvy effect—blouson tops, soft shirring, gathers, ruffles, and flowing lines. Vertical lines tend to make you look straighter. Don't wear anything too tight—you'll look flatter. You might want to try a slightly padded bra to round out your bosom, if that's how you'd like to see yourself. Or you can revel in the fact that almost everything you wear looks fabulous, with or without a bra.

LARGE WAIST: When you wear a belt, wear an open jacket, vest, or sweater with it to create the illusion of a waist. Dresses with high or low waistlines are perfect for you. Look for pants with elastic in the back of the waist only—that creates a clean, easy-fitting look in front. Pull-on pants with full elastic add too much bulk at the waist. Avoid wide belts.

LONG OR SHORT WAIST: These are subtle problems that usually result in poor fitting clothes. Some of the problems can be alleviated by wearing separates. Pants pose the biggest problem for short-waisted women. The easiest solution is to wear overblouses or jackets. Long-waisted women need to create a shorter line from shoulder to waist, which can be done by wearing wide belts, printed or horizontally striped tops, large collars, or short vests layered over lean sweaters. The long-waisted woman can also exaggerate the long line by wearing lean, tucked-in sweaters and tops accented with skinny little belts.

LARGE HIPS: The secret is to balance wide hips with a broad shoulder line. The current trend toward shoulder pads is the perfect solution—not the severe, Joan Crawford look that her costume designer, Adrian, made famous in the forties, but a softer, subtler look that adds just enough width at the shoulders to make the hips look proportionate. An elongated jacket or cardigan sweater will also help slim the hip. If you wear your jacket open, add a belt at the waist to create some interest above the hip line. Avoid shoulder bags, which ride on your hip; a clutch bag is better.

THE LARGE DERRIERE: Invest in a three-way mirror so that you always know how you look coming *and* going. You may be surprised to know that dresses look better on you than skirts, since a longer line from shoulder to hem seems to deemphasize the rear end. Keep stockings and shoes in the same tone as the dress. Avoid definite waistlines, although an elasticized blouson waist can be very flattering, especially if your upper torso is small in proportion to your derriere. When wearing a two-tone outfit, keep brighter colors on top, darker or neutral colors on the bottom. Don't give up on pants—just make sure they're not too tight. Wear longer vests or blouses to softly cover those protruding buns. Check your rear-view mirror before you go out to make sure the line is smooth.

THE SMALL DERRIERE: Take solace in the fact that many women wish they had your problem. Then look for those marvelous gathered skirts and trousers that look best on women like you. Wear hip-length sweaters and jackets— those elongated blouson styles were meant for you. Jackets and dresses with peplums add a bit of fluff in the right spot. When swimsuit shopping, you can take one of two approaches: buy one of the softly skirted suits, or go for one of the sleek, very high-thigh bikinis that will make you look "all leg."

POUCHY TUMMY: Soft, flowing clothes that float over the body minimize your problem; tight clothing will emphasize it. Trousers with soft pleats at the waist add just enough fullness to deemphasize your bulge. Dresses or skirts with dropped waistlines and slightly gathered skirts are also flattering. If you like the look of a slim skirt, wear a jacket or sweater with a peplum that hides the abdomen. Also, a body-stocking will often give just enough support to flatten a tummy pouch.

The All-Important Et Cetera

As every fashion specialist will tell you, accessories are what add an extra bit of dash to your wardrobe. They create your personal style—they say, "This is me." Designer Bill Blass asserts that the accessories actually make the outfit. "I think what you wear between your neck and your knee are not as important as the belt, shoes, and the bag." Liz Claiborne concurs: "I believe in spending a little more on shoes than on individual pieces of clothing, and if you live in a winter climate, you must invest in a few good pairs of boots, as well." Geoffrey Beene adds, "A collection of accessories is essential to a basic wardrobe. Through the coloration of scarves, jewelry, handbags, and shoes, one is able to change the look of so-called basics."

Generally speaking, what these designers are telling us is this: Anyone can buy a white silk blouse and a pair of black gabardine trousers. A woman who has a sense of style might add a red taffeta pussycat bow at her neck and carry a purple and red tapestry clutchbag. Another might toss a large turquoise and pink paisley shawl over one shoulder and cinch her waist with the belt she borrowed from her pink silk cocktail dress. Still another woman might wear the turquoise squash blossom necklace she inherited from her grandmother and leave her blouse unbuttoned to the waist. All make their own statement.

Image consultant Alayne Harris explains that accessories such as belts, scarves, and jewelry are an excellent way to wear a fashion color that otherwise would not look good on you. If olive is "in" but it looks terrible on you, try an olive scarf tied under the collar of your red blouse, or an olive belt. Your wardrobe gets a fresh look, and your skin doesn't look washed out. Fashion coordinator Andrea Sells notes that choosing an imaginative accessory that expresses something unique about your personality is far more desirable than spending a fortune on a fad. Her favorite example? "I'd much rather see someone wearing a classic Mickey Mouse watch then a *de rigueur* Rolex, or worse yet—a copy of the Rolex. Wearing fad items or copies of fine things only points out one's insecurities. Being unique is far more important than following the fashion herd."

There are two approaches to accessory collecting. One is the classic approach: buying timeless jewelry, scarves, handbags, shoes, and belts that you know will bring you years of pleasure. The other, equally expressive technique is to invest in inexpensive trendy items that follow the current mood of fashion while still expressing your personal taste. If you tire of things quickly and like to be in fashion, this could be the route for you.

Posture—Stand Up for Yourself

Diana Vreeland, one of the world's foremost fashion authorities, told me that beauty has much to do with the extension of the neck, extension of the arms, extension of the back, extension of the legs, and a very light step. She's right. Your posture has everything to say about you. If you're down or depressed, you tend to slouch. If you're tired, you slump. If you're insecure, your posture takes on a curve. Luckily, you can teach your posture to say what you want it to—you can train it to express your self-confidence and say the right thing all the time. Here's how: Straighten your spine, keep shoulders back, tuck your tummy in, align your hips, keep your head up—all those things drill sergeants and your mom have said so often.

Again, your mirror is your constant source of honesty. Take off all your clothes and face your body straight on. Do your shoulders slope down? Is your chest concave? Do you bunch up around your waist? Is one hip higher than the other? Now look at yourself from the side. Does your head jut forward? Do your shoulders curve in? Does your spine curve toward your protruding belly? Do your buttocks stick out to compensate for that curving spine?

If so, you're not alone. Many people have terrible posture. But the good news is that you can improve yours just by thinking about it—well, almost.

A POSTURE-PERFECT EXERCISE

You'll have to exert a little energy, too. Choose a day when you can afford to devote needed attention to yourself. When you get up that morning, check out your posture in the mirror. As you look at each part of your body, consciously attempt to straighten it, all the while breathing rhythmically. Place your head and neck in line with your spine. Shrug your shoulders, roll them around a bit, and let them relax naturally. If they curve forward, use your shoulder muscles to pull them back slightly, which will automatically pull up your sunken chest. (Are you breathing evenly?) Next, tuck your buttocks under and in while flattening your tummy. This will align your spine. Now, as if someone had suspended your head from a string, maintain this alignment while you walk around the room.

Now, lay down on your back on a firm surface, attempting to maintain the same body alignment. Push your spine as close to the floor as possible. Bend your knees and feel your spine naturally push closer to the ground. Close your eyes and take six very deep breaths. Feel your abdomen and lungs fill up and expand as you breathe in; feel them slowly deflate as you exhale. With your legs still bent and with your arms straight out in front of you, slowly curl up into a sitting position. Align your body and straighten your legs. Sit up as tall as possible, with your arms extending forward. Tucking your chin toward your chest, bend your body forward, hands reaching toward your toes. Slowly stretch your spine.

Stand up and realign yourself. Take a warm shower, all the while practicing your alignment. Finish with a blast of cold water. Dry off, concentrating on each part of your body as you blot the water. Are you maintaining your new alignment? Proceed with the rest of your day's activities, but recheck your body alignment every fifteen minutes. By day's end, you will have rediscovered some muscles you forgot you had. Take another warm shower, letting the water beat on your tired muscles between your shoulders and in the back of your neck. Try to sleep on your back or side with your knees bent.

This exercise helps to build body awareness. The best part is that your mirror gives you constant reinforcement. When your body is properly aligned, you instantly look better. The longer you practice good posture, the faster it becomes second nature to you. Practice constantly, whether sitting, standing, walking, or relaxing. Soon good posture will be a fact of life.

About Those Not-So-Instant Changes

LET A DENTIST FILL YOU IN

Unattractive teeth can ruin an otherwise pretty smile. With all the technological advances in modern dentistry, many of which have extraordinary cosmetic advantages, there's almost no reason for going around with a mouth full of anything but pearly whites. Of course, nothing is a substitute for regular brushing, flossing, and those twice-yearly professional checkups, but there's nothing to say you can't go to the dentist more frequently and come out looking prettier.

Consider the fact that no one is too old for orthodontia. Realigning the position of your teeth and improving your bite can be done at just about any age. According to Beverly Hills dentist Dr. Robert Smith, there are clear braces with plastic brackets and white wires, which are only slightly visible. Other forms of braces can be placed behind the teeth if the mouth needs to be expanded. One type is a removable retainer called a crozat, which can be worn all the time or just at night, depending on the work to be done.

If you have a space between your teeth that you'd like corrected, you should know about a removable cap that you can pop in place whenever you need it. Known as a "flipper," this kind of cosmetic appliance usually comes attached to a retainer and can cover one or more teeth. Because these caps are removable, your own teeth are not permanently affected—no grinding, filing, or extractions. Nancy Wheeler's before and after shots, shown here, show how a flipper changes her appearance.

If your teeth are stained, consider two options. One is bleaching the teeth; the other is a relatively new method in which the teeth are actually painted with a composite material that adheres to the natural surface of the teeth. Dr. Smith explains that bleaching is a process in which a specially developed dental bleaching solution is applied directly to the teeth. Dr. Mardy Doyle, a Los Angeles dentist, advocates this method of tooth whitening. After the composite material is painted on the teeth, a zap of ultraviolet light sets it. One treatment lasts for three to five years, according to Dr. Doyle.

Both dentists agree that neither method is a substitute for proper brushing, which can help to prevent most dental stains.

Finally, you might want to think about bonding, a procedure that is gaining more and more attention these days. Bonding is a process wherein the natural surface of the tooth is etched with acid and then coated or extended with a composite plastic. Dr. Doyle takes the process one step further and applies a thin plastic cover, or veneer, to the tooth or teeth, sealing the entire tooth. In the event the veneer "cap" is accidentally broken, the natural tooth underneath remains unharmed. According to Dr. Doyle, "The veneer cap duplicates the natural tooth exactly and retains its appearance without staining for years. Time in the dentist's chair is minimal, and there is no pain. Up to six teeth can be capped in about two hours, and the cost is far less than conventional capping."

WHAT TO DO ABOUT WRINKLES

Nothing removes wrinkles; but there are a few procedures that might interest you if you care to minimize them.

For instance, injectible collagen can plump up and smooth out wrinkles so the skin doesn't sag and the lines aren't as pronounced. It was approved by the FDA in July of 1981. Since then, it has been used on many patients to fill out

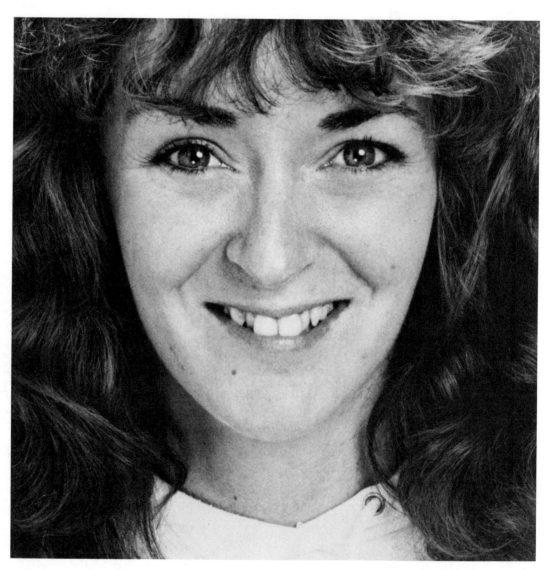

Nancy Wheeler

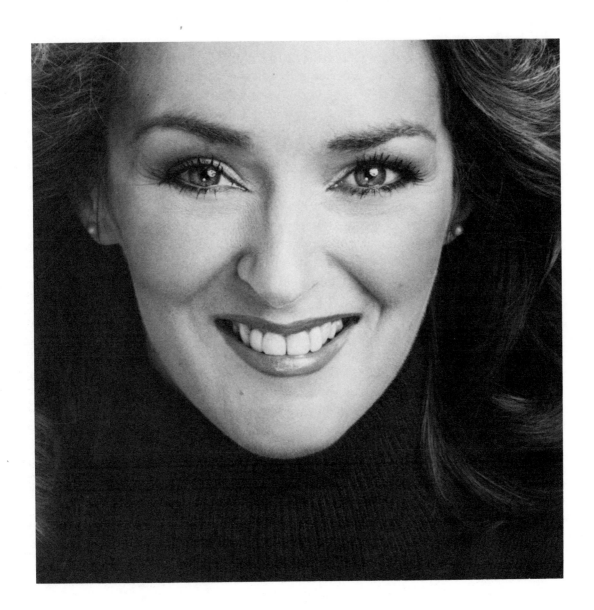

smile lines and the vertical frown lines that frequently appear between the eyebrows. These implants are composed of 35 percent collagen and 65 percent saline solution for fine lines, and 65 percent collagen and 35 percent saline for deep furrows.

At the time of injection, a line or depressed scar may be completely plumped up and smoothed out, but within a few days the saline solution is absorbed. Therefore, repeated injections are sometimes necessary to implant enough collagen to achieve desired results. After it is injected, the collagen begins to act exactly like the natural collagen that is a normal part of the connective tissue in the human body. Over time the injected collagen breaks down, like the natural collagen, and is flushed out of the system. Because of this process, further injections may be needed.

Medical scientists in America have not as yet given the nod to acupuncture as a way to treat wrinkled skin, since there has been no documented, scientific proof that it works. However, acupuncture is a traditional form of Chinese medicine that originated more than five thousand years ago, and as the oldest form of medicine known to man, it has a distinguished following. Dr. Steven Rosenblatt of Los Angeles employs both laser and metal needles in his acupuncture therapy, and claims that "acupuncture activates energies in the face to regain muscular tone." He goes on to explain, "You are born with certain patterns in which wrinkles will form. Deepening and increasing lines can be halted with acupuncture by stimulating the underlying musculature, increasing its elasticity." No one claims that the lift from acupuncture is permanent, but some skin specialists do agree that wrinkles can be temporarily smoothed and further wrinkling may be slowed.

Many women swear by facial exercises for reducing wrinkles, noting that these above-the-neck calisthenics keep faces firm and chins taut. Dermatologist Dr. Arnold Klein insists that "wrinkles only come from degeneration of the skin as a result of sun exposure. They do not come from weakened facial muscles. Facial exercises aren't going to get rid of wrinkles. Staying out of the sun will." But Gerald Schneider, a former New York chiropractor who makes his living massaging some of the most beautiful faces in the world—Morgan Fairchild, Goldie Hawn, Leslie Ann Warren, Mary Ann Mobley, to name a few—disagrees. "There are no empty spaces in the body. The skin is attached to a layer of muscle. The skin moves with the muscles. Keep the muscles firm and you will improve the look of the face." In addition to frequent hand massages, which Schneider himself adminsters, he also suggests some easy, do-at-home exercises:

- To tone facial muscles, start under your chin and, using your middle fingers, stroke your muscles in a rapid but gentle circular motion moving upward toward the cheeks for five to ten minutes each day.

- To combat lines in the neck, point the chin up and out, then repeat the circular massage with your middle fingers.

Finally, dermabrasion can be very effective on surface wrinkles, but anyone who decides to undergo dermabrasion or a chemical peel should understand that these are medical procedures not to be taken lightly. Dark skin does not seem to respond as well to the treatments and, in some cases, even women with fair skin find that their skin tones are not even after dermabrasion or a chemical peel. Consult a dermatologist and/or plastic surgeon about both procedures before getting your heart set on miraculous results.

FACIAL HAIR

There are several ways to remedy the situation, the most effective—in my estimation—being waxing. It's inexpensive, whether you do it at home or have it professionally done in a salon. It lasts three to four weeks and leaves your skin very soft, with no rough stubble when the hair grows back. Waxing over a long period of time can eventually kill enough of the hair follicle to prevent further regrowth. Shaving is not recommended for a woman's face, since the stubble is dark and grows back quickly. Bleaching facial hair is another alternative.

Electrolysis, on the other hand, is the only known permanent means of hair removal. However, sometimes the follicle of the hair is so strong that the electrical impulse from the needle only weakens the hair growth, but does not fully destroy it. "Regrowth continues and, in some cases, it can take up to a year to completely remove hair," explains electrologist Tami Iguchi.

Lucy Peters, a New York electrologist, worked with two doctors to develop an insulated bulbous probe, which, she says, permanently destroys the hair's follicle while protecting the skin from damage or unnecessary discomfort.

As for body hair, Tami Iguchi notes that hair on the body seems to be easier to remove permanently by electrolysis, and she theorizes that perhaps it's because the sun does not stimulate hair growth in those areas. Since the face is constantly exposed, the hair follicles are over-stimulated and more difficult to inhibit. Another method, waxing, is quick and can last up to a month. Bleaching also can be effective. Home kits for bleaching hair on the upper lip, arms, and bikini line are available, or you can mix your own solution by combining two parts of 20-volume hydrogen peroxide (less than $1 for sixteen fluid ounces) with one part of Clairol's Clairolite 4 (about $3); both are available at beauty supply stores. Leave the mixture on for at least five minutes the first time, and check for lightness.

In the next several pages, you'll see before and after photos of many women. Many have had their images changed merely by a change of clothes, following the concepts discussed in the beginning of this chapter. I've included a wide variety of uniquely beautiful women in this chapter because they each have something to contribute to the concepts we've discussed.

JOETTE LAFOND

At five feet ten inches, size 16 Joette LaFond was trapped, like so many other large women, into thinking that she looked best in pull-on pants and an overblouse. Carole Shaw, editor of *Big Beautiful Woman* magazine, calls this the "fat lady costume," an outfit large women wear to fit the role society has established for them. Unfortunately, in most cases, pull-on pants and a shapeless blouse are the least flattering thing a woman can choose.

Joette's new fashion image breaks all the old rules. Her waist is belted. Her white blouse is not only ruffled, but tucked in, too. Her slim corduroy trousers are brightly colored. Notice, too, her ballet slippers and gold Art Nouveau earrings.

Once we used those fashion tricks to enhance Joette's large but well-proportioned figure, we applied makeup that accentuated her high cheek-bones and emphasized and elongated her dark, lovely eyes.

All in all, Joette's new look gives her style and a look of comfort with her own image. She's ready for her next adventure.

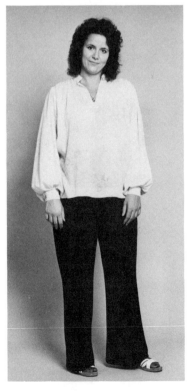 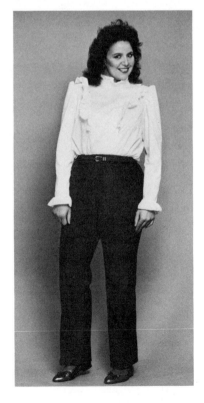

Joette LaFond

ZAIDA BEDELL

Like so many homemakers, Zaida Bedell decided to go back to work after many years at home with family responsibilities. Now she wanted a new sophisticated professional image that would match her enthusiasm about this new phase in her life.

At five-foot-two, Zaida explained that she'd like to look taller, but her before outfit does just about everything to make her look shorter. The long poncho, with its bold black and white plaid, is overpowering. A wide belt cuts her in half, defeating the possibility of a long, vertical look. Her cuffed pants shorten her legs, especially when paired with flat white shoes that draw attention.

The solution for Zaida was easy, especially since she had a well-proportioned figure to start with. A long, lean pantsuit, all one color, with a sophisticated contrasting blouse. The vertical line of the suit makes her look taller immediately. Her shoes, with two-inch heels, match her suit, thus continuing the line. Wearing her hair up adds the illusion of more height.

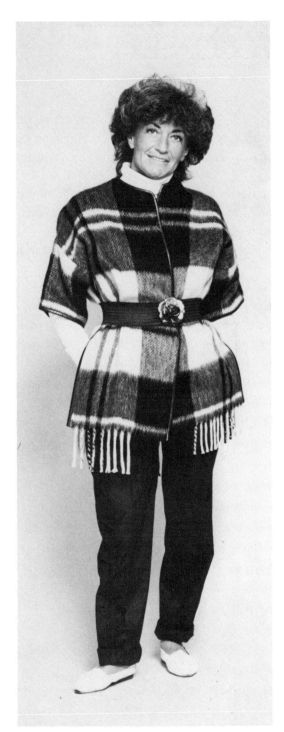
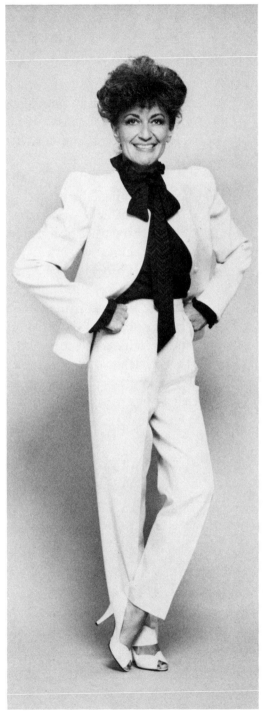

Zaida Bedell

ANGELA GOSSETT

Angela Gossett is a sales representative for a line of women's clothing, so she has to look her fashionable best every day. Her problem is that her body is thick from her shoulders to her stomach. But her hips are fairly slim, and she has nice legs.

With the busy floral pattern and complicated, bulky silhouette of her before clothing, she looks top heavy. The full sleeve adds too much volume, and the neckline has too many tiers. Her pumps look bulky because of the two-toned toe and thick heel. The skirt is just a bit too long to accentuate the lovely curve of her calf.

Angela benefits from a body stocking, an undergarment that includes bra and panties in one and provides gentle, all-over control. A slim, long dress in a soft, silk jacquard pattern establishes one long line from shoulder to hemline. The high-heeled shoe gives Angela a bit more height. The soft tie at the neck and the large hat switches focus from her bustline to her face.

Angela's makeup emphasizes her beautiful almond-shaped eyes, and I used highlighter and contour shadows to define her cheeks and give her nose a narrower appearance. Angela's confident smile testifies to her feeling about the new look.

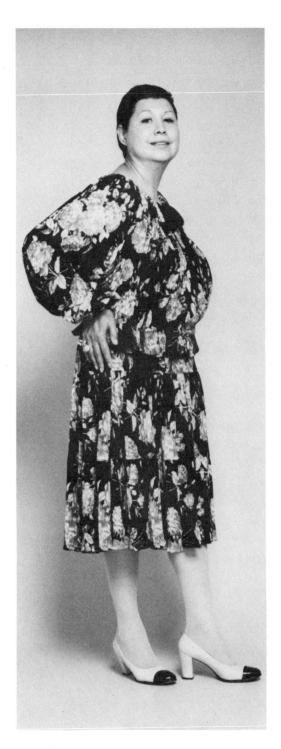
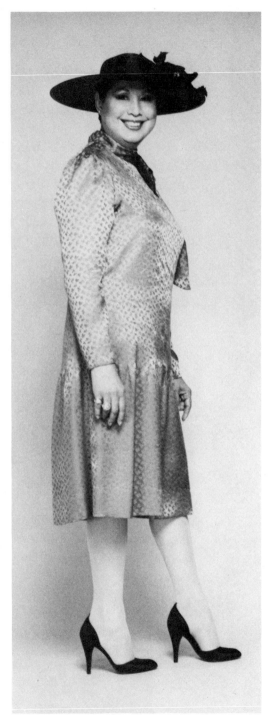

Angela Gossett

B. COURTENAY LEIGH

B. Courtenay Leigh, a large-size model and a successful actress/singer, didn't lose an ounce, but she looks slimmer, more self-confident and happier because of a few simple changes. First, notice her posture. In her after photo she has her shoulders back, which helps lift her rib cage. Her blouse flatters her in many ways, too. First, her round shoulders get a straighter, broader look from the large collar, and the slightly lowered round neckline makes her neck appear longer than it actually is. The black trim on the blouse tapers to a slenderizing *V*, and the soft, loose fabric is both flattering and feminine. Piling

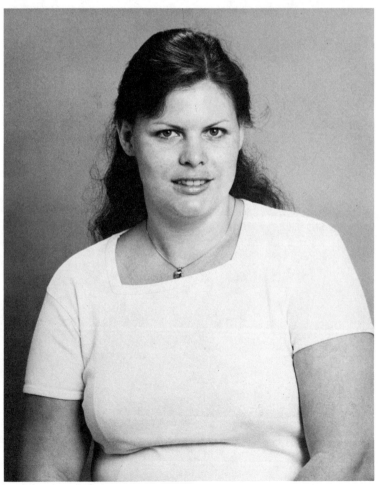

B. Courtenay Leigh

her hair on top of her head elongates the look of her face and neck, accenting her high cheekbones.

When I applied Courtenay's makeup, I concentrated on giving her cheekbones more prominence by using highlighter above them and by applying contour shadow high and under the cheekbones, at the temples, along the jawline, and under the chin, all of which worked to slim her face.

Afterwards, when Courtenay looked in the mirror, she actually seemed to have a glowing self-confidence that wasn't apparent before her instant makeover.

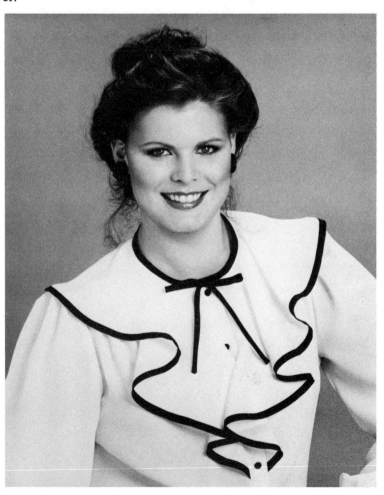

ELLEN MILLER

Though Ellen Miller had spent a fortune on a beautiful ribbon knit sweater and on an expensive and equally lovely belt, neither investment was profitable. They don't flatter her. Because she has a large bustline, a tight-fitting sweater accentuates the fullness. With a bold belt, she looks like her breasts are right on top of her waist. She also needs proper support from a better-fitted bra.

Ellen likes the idea of wearing a light-colored top, which brightens her face, with a dark skirt. Lightweight fabrics and soft, flowing silhouettes are more flattering to her figure than the heavily textured combination of light and dark she wears in her before photo. In her after photo, Ellen wears a minimizer bra, which helps control her ample bustline. Wearing a loose-fitting white silk blouse with dolman sleeves and a smooth, slim-lined black silk skirt with white side panels gives Ellen a long, slim vertical line when teamed with dark hose and shoes. Her geometric earrings and swept-back hairstyle draw attention to her face.

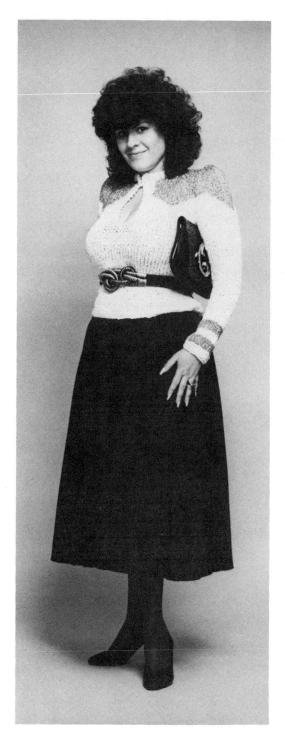 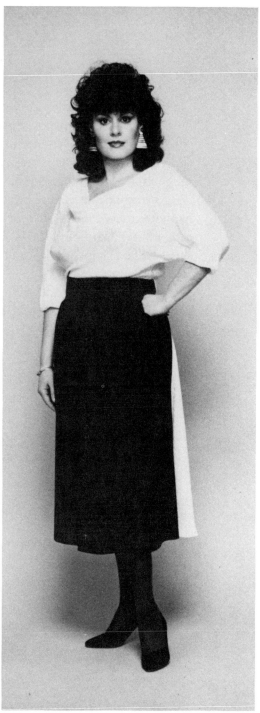

Ellen Miller

ROZ WEINER

Roz Weiner, mother of two, has a slim waist, a narrow torso, and large hips and thighs. She's not a prime candidate for white slacks; light-colored pants add pounds. Her bright-colored camisole emphasizes her narrow top and contrasts glaringly with her wide bottom. Her large shoulder bag adds width exactly where she doesn't need it—at her hip line.

To create balance, Roz wears a puffed-sleeve, padded-shoulder blouse for her after photo. Her dropped-waist skirt highlights her slim waist and camouflages her figure flaws with gentle fullness. Dark-toned hosiery and shoes make her look taller, and the clutch bag and large onyx earrings draw attention upward.

I used highlighter and contour shadows on Roz's narrow face to give it a wider look, all of which works to add proportion to her overall image.

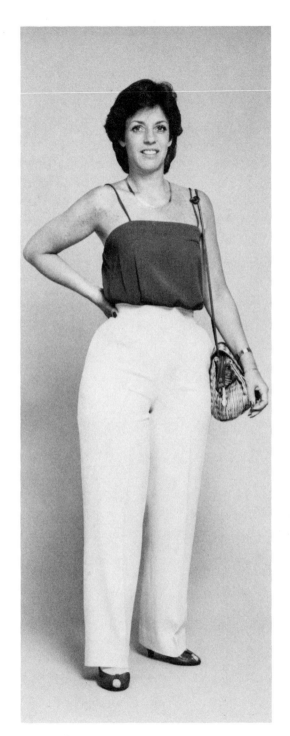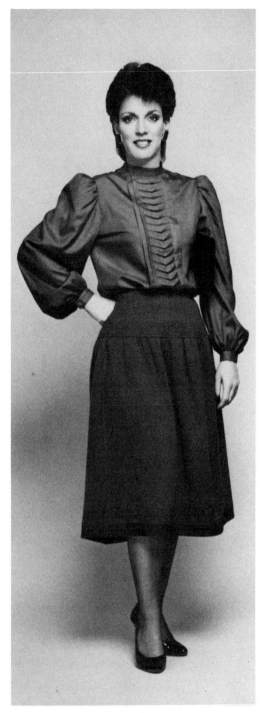

Roz Weiner

PHYLLIS DILLER

Phyllis Diller has spent her life making people laugh. People are usually laughing so hard that they forget what a lovely and intelligent human being she is under those egg-beater hairdos and bizarre costumes. Phyllis describes herself like this: "I've built a very stylized character, and I'm very proud of it. But it is certainly not me in person. My outlandish clothing and the fright wigs are my work clothes—happy Halloween! I have never felt ugly. I felt that I could be improved, but I knew I had inner beauty. My mother saw to that. She told me that inner beauty was important. That's when I first suspected that I was not Liz Taylor."

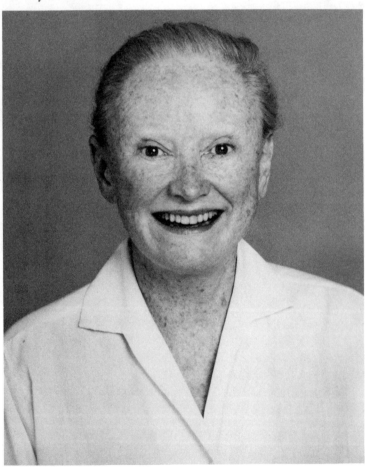

Phyllis Diller

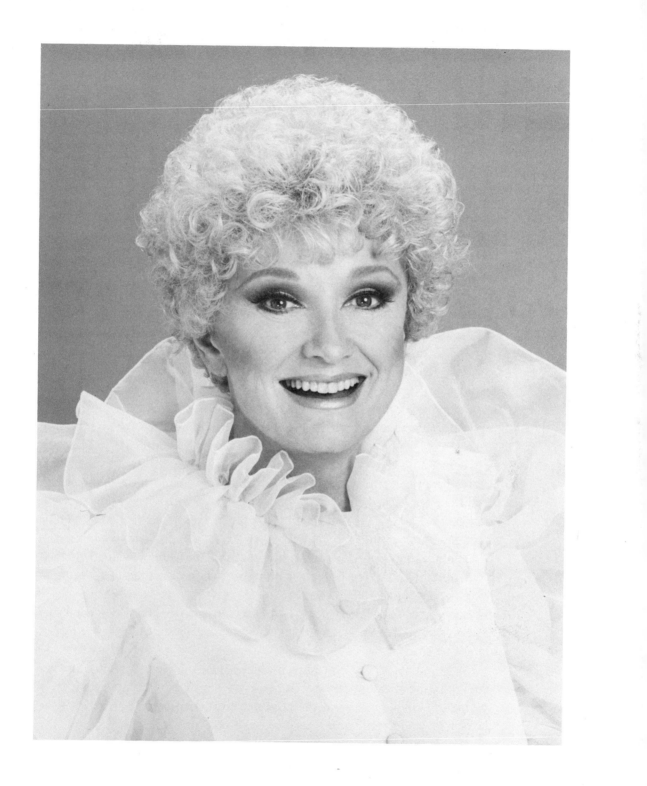

It wasn't until she was thirty-four years old that Phyllis decided to give up being a journalist and ad copy writer to become a comedienne. The mother of five, in a period when women's liberation was still equated with the suffragettes, she was scared of making such a major change in her life, but she remembers knowing she wouldn't be happy until she took the chance.

"Some people are afraid forever. I was such a fearful person that eventually I couldn't do anything. I would turn away from a project if I got a dirty look. Then I got hold of a book, *The Magic of Believing*, by Claude Bristol, and it struck a chord. I realized that fear is a dumb thing that makes you ill and keeps you from ever performing properly. It keeps you from being a success and makes you difficult to be with."

When she turned thirty-seven, Phyllis appeared at the Purple Onion Club in San Francisco, where she ranted and raved about being a housewife—and the rest is history. As she became more and more self-confident, she started making more changes. Her divorce was one of the first.

"It takes courage to change anything. The slightest bit of change can upset people. But I think a good divorce is better than a bad marriage. You have to be able to give up some kind of security to gain in every area of life. I've tried to change for the better in every area of my life—even my looks.

"Before I became successful, I didn't have the money to improve my physical appearance. Slowly, I had my teeth straightened, then I bought contact lenses, and finally, I bought a new face, which I adore. My old face got me where I am—it was a fine face, but it was not a pretty face to live with. Before I had my face job—including nose and everything—I got all the 'witch' parts. In fact, it was when I was playing a witch on television and saw myself at home on my own TV set that I realized I needed a new face. (*Puhleeze!* People might have been eating!)

"I immediately called a plastic surgeon and told him I wanted to look rested, not different. He told me it would cost five thousand dollars—and that was only the *estimate*!

"Everybody said a new face would wreck my career. Did they think my career was built on a broken nose? I knew it wasn't. It was built on hard work and honest study."

Phyllis actually shaves off her eyebrows because they're so low. Because her hair is thin, she always wears one of her many wigs when she's working.

Though Phyllis wears heavy stage makeup when she's performing, she relaxes with a clean, glowing, no-makeup look. "I'm not going to put my makeup on to go to the grocery or to take the dog to the vet. I may put makeup on the dog—but not on me! I surround myself with beauty at all times. I have a beautiful home, beautiful clothes, and whatever else makes me feel beautiful. It's up to you to build yourself up, you know."

Phyllis's makeup centers around her well-spaced, hazel eyes. Highlighter applied above the cheekbones creates an illusion of "lifting" the eyes. I used plum shadow in the crease of the eyelids blended up toward the brow; light pink shadow on the lid and brow bone; slate blue shadow in the outer triangles at the corners of her eyes; and charcoal pencil eye liner on her top and bottom lids, smudged slightly. A strip of artificial lashes on the upper lid and two coats of black mascara completed the eye makeup application. Since Phyllis had no brows, we created them using silvery beige and light brown eyebrow pencils applied with short strokes in the direction in which the brows would normally grow.

Richard Bradshaw styled Phyllis's soft blond wig for her after photo. Finally, a soft, ruffled neckline frames her beautiful face and glowing personality.

THE REVEREND TERRY COLE-WHITTAKER

My life changed when I met the Reverend Terry Cole-Whittaker, the "guru of entertaining enlightenment." She's a radiant, absolutely beautiful person, beaming with health and vitality and bubbling with good humor. Terry believes that "you can giggle your way to the top, allow yourself to be physically beautiful and abundantly prosperous, while still pursuing the ineffable goals of spiritual advancement.

"Beauty is letting go of the need to *be* beautiful according to the standards of the world. Accept yourself, then out of accepting yourself, be as beautiful as you can. I think of everyone—including myself—as an art expression of God. Every art expression is unique. Every person is beautiful. What is ugly is the fear and anger that people lock in their consciousness and in their bodies.

"The more a person loves himself, the more he allows himself to be beautiful.

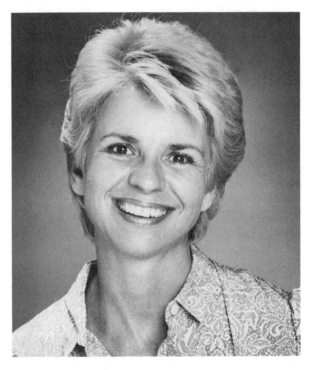

Rev. Terry Cole-Whittaker

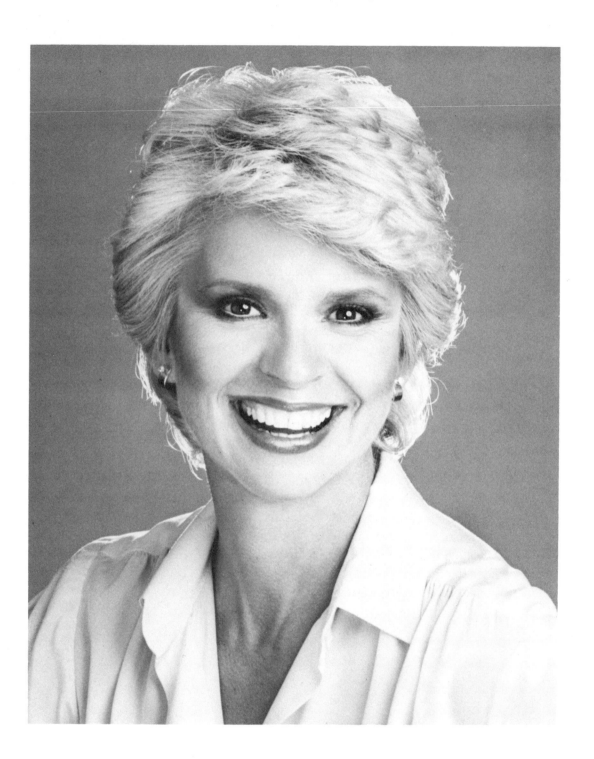

"You cannot *become* beautiful. You *are* beautiful within. You must allow that beauty to come out. When we become comfortable with ourselves, we appreciate our own unique beauty. People sometimes think it's not okay to be beautiful or prosperous or successful. That's all part of our old negative religious training. We have the freedom to choose what our presentation of ourselves is—how we want to look. We have the freedom to be the art expression that we are. We should express that fully."

A former beauty contest winner, Terry feels that she looks best in clothing that makes a presentation of excellence, beauty, and prosperity, not necessarily high fashion. She also believes that the colors she wears have an impact on her life. She loves tans and ivories, but feels people respond well to her when she wears peach tones. She'll usually wear bright yellow if she's feeling down.

"Yellow gives me a lot of energy. But if I want to give a powerful message, I wear red. I usually don't wear black. Green is very healing. I remember one period when I was going through a lot of body work and needed healing. I bought an emerald green running suit—and it healed my body."

Terry's hair is coarse and straight. Stylist Raphael San Nicolas accented it with various blond highlights. She has it trimmed every two and a half weeks and conditions with Nexus Keraphix and a placenta treatment after every shampoo. She uses a curling iron for a soft, casual curl in her layered hair.

Terry keeps up an incredible pace, managing to devote her attention to her humanitarian goals. She writes her own sermons and has just completed her new book, *How to Have More in a Have-Not World*. She has developed a worldwide television ministry and still finds time to jog four times a week, do aerobic exercise three times a week, and be a loving wife and mother. And there are still enough hours in the day to keep herself looking terrific. How does she do it all? "There isn't anyone who doesn't want to be beautiful, healthy, happy, wealthy, loved, and successful. If they say they don't, they're denying it, only because they don't know they can be. When you want things badly enough, you find ways to accomplish all of them."

GERI JEWELL

Sometimes people in the audience don't know how to laugh at comedienne Geri Jewell's jokes. After all, they reason, you aren't supposed to laugh at people with cerebral palsy. They don't realize that Geri isn't uptight about being disabled and that, more than anything, she wants them to laugh *with* her.

"Being a comedienne has allowed me to be an adult, a child, to be funny, serious, and most of all, accepted. When I was in high school, I thought that no one would want to date me because I was disabled. I only wore corduroys, T-shirts, and Wallabees. That was the extent of my wardrobe. I didn't date until I was twenty-three. But my career gave me self-confidence. I'm not afraid to try things. The turning point was when I realized that I had to accomplish things to please myself, not to prove anything to other people."

With that thought foremost in her mind, Geri stopped letting her physical disability limit her ambition or minimize her potential. Before long, producer Norman Lear "discovered" her when she performed at a banquet sponsored by the California Governor's Committee for Employment of the Handicapped. He was impressed with her ability to use humor to foster a better understanding of cerebral palsy among a non-handicapped audience.

Geri, who now makes frequent appearances as Geri on Lear's "The Facts of Life," says it took her twenty-six years to realize that she was pretty. "My sister Gloria, a model, is gorgeous, so I was always comparing myself to her. I had to learn to love my inner self, and that love began to shine through. I finally realized that we all have our own individual beauty and we express it in our own ways. I was blessed with a sense of humor, and even though many negative people told me I'd never make it as a comedienne, I never had any doubt that I would."

Today Geri dresses to suit her mood. A devotee of what she calls "funky clothes," she says she wears slacks most often. "But if I'm feeling sexy, I'll wear a satin blouse and slacks. I wear makeup now, too. It used to take me hours to apply it, but I can do it well now in about fifteen minutes." She keeps her hair short and enjoys the simplicity of it. For her after photo, stylist Doug Martin added volume to her hair with a curling iron and separated her permed curls with a vent brush.

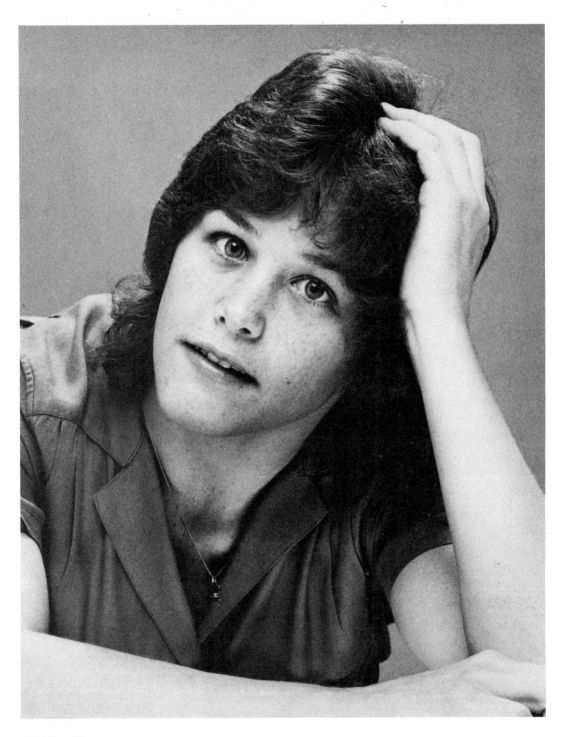

Geri Jewell

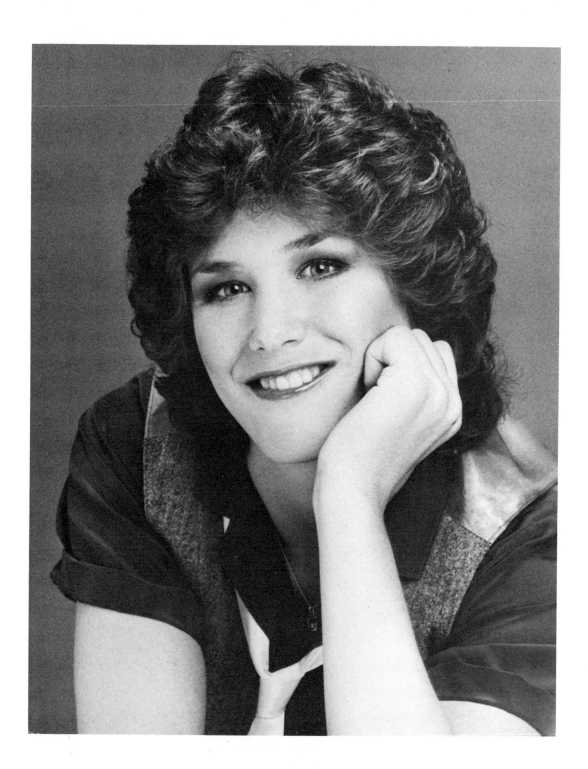

BETTY GARRETT

Betty Garrett has a reputation for being a joy to work with, whether she's in films, on stage or on television's "Laverne and Shirley." I asked about her secrets for getting along with people. "I have no secrets at all," she told me matter-of-factly. "I love my work, I only take projects that I know I can have a good time doing, I'm not a competitive person, and I hate backbiting. I'm just a basically happy person."

Betty welcomes her gray hair. She feels it adds interest and glamour to what might otherwise be considered "mousey" hair. She usually wears it up to show off those marvelous cheekbones.

When applying Betty's makeup, I used concealer on her eyelids and highlighter at the inner corners to make them seem wider spaced. Concealer around her nostrils camouflages some of the lines ʌre. I used shadows and eye liners to make Betty's lovely round eyes appear a bit larger, and lip liner applied outside her natural lip line, on the upper lip only, gives her mouth a fuller, luscious look.

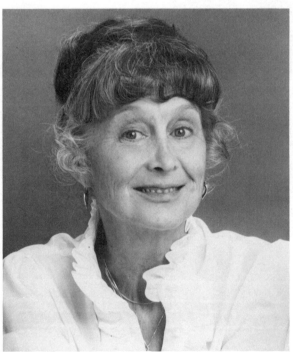

Betty Garrett

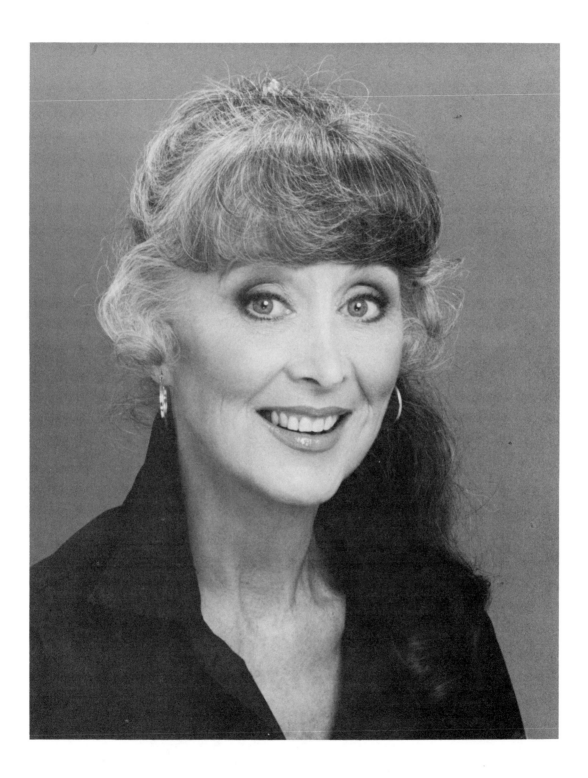

ELLA TOWNS

When I first discovered Ella Towns, now a top model, I knew she had potential, but she tended to overdress, she wore bright blue eye shadow, her brows needed tweezing, and she lacked self-confidence. She wanted a make-over, and I suggested that she take some dance classes to firm up and become more aware of her body. She also learned to simplify her wardrobe.

After her makeover and hours of work in front of my camera, she became more comfortable and self-assured. I could see she was turning into a gorgeous, dedicated professional. I knew she was ready to meet the head of one of the world's top modeling agencies, Nina Blanchard. I arranged a meeting, and within moments of their first encounter, Nina offered her a contract with the agency. In a short time, Ella had become one of the top models in Los Angeles and had signed a contract to be the Salem Slim Lights girl.

Ella has charisma—that elusive ability to attract others. Nina explained it to me this way: "I don't believe that beauty is just in the eye of the beholder. There are more pleasing faces than others, but even a very beautiful woman can become unattractive by the way she moves her face and what happens in

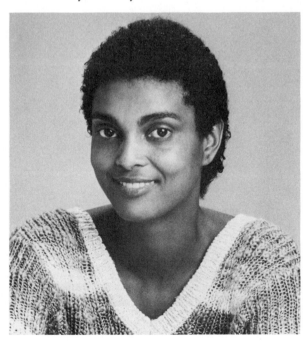

Ella Towns

her eyes. In the same way, a less attractive woman can be magnificent by what she communicates."

I used a mocha-toned cream foundation on Ella's flawless skin. Since her round, full cheeks tend to hide her cheekbones, I used a touch of highlighter above her cheekbones and in the areas immediately under the hollows of her cheeks to create an angular effect. Dark brown contour shadow exaggerates the hollows of the cheeks, and shadow at the temples narrows her forehead. These cosmetic improvements only work to enhance Ella's great smile and sensual image.

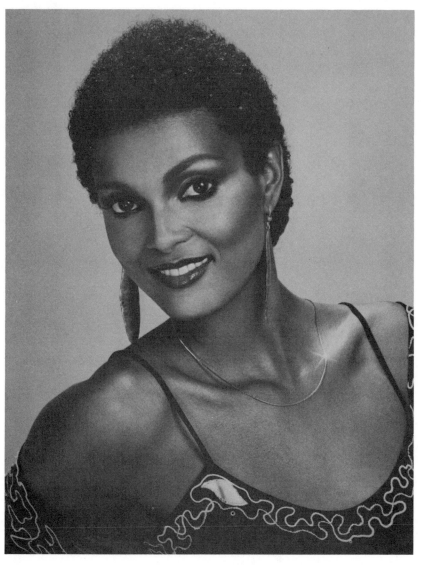

JANIS PAIGE

Musical comedy star Janis Paige is a joy to be around, with constant positive energy flowing. I asked her how she defines beauty and found that her explanation reflected her own inner loveliness. "Beauty is individuality and self-esteem. It's quietly feeling good about yourself without being narcissistic. It's taking responsibility for yourself."

When Janis's husband died, she says she learned to be more self-reliant. "I realized that it's extremely difficult to depend on yourself, but it is a wonderful way to live. I learned to be kinder—to myself, because no one else was going to pamper me anymore."

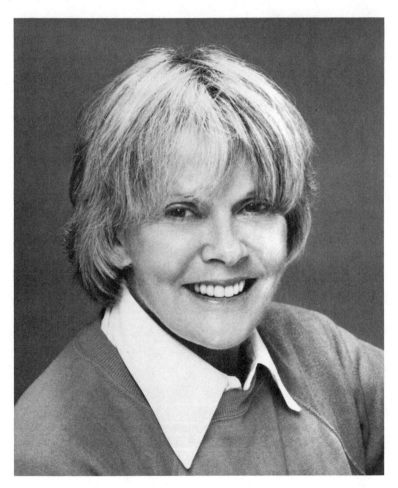

Janis Paige

Janis learned that exercise can be wonderful therapy. She does it often, sometimes with two- or five-pound weights on her ankles. This five-foot-five-and-a-half-inch beauty attributes her flawless complexion to at-home facials, a mixture of avocado, bananas, and yogurt applied regularly.

Janis has a wonderful face that features large, round green eyes, even skin tones, high cheekbones, and nicely shaped lips. The makeup I used for her after photo only enhanced these wonderful characteristics. Eric Root used his fingers to style Janis's hair after using a few hot rollers.

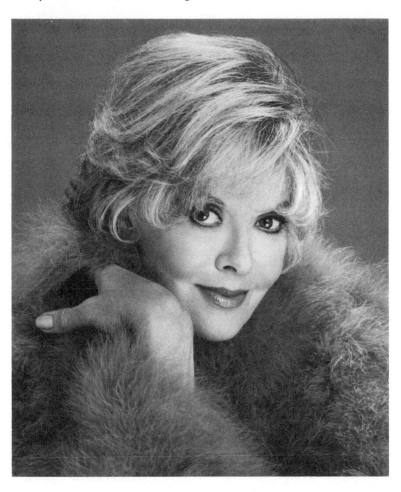

GLORIA DE HAVEN

At five feet two inches and 110 pounds, veteran actress Gloria De Haven says, "I can't always keep up with fashion because I'm too short for many of the trends. I try to be contemporary, but ultimately, I dress to flatter my figure. I prefer soft, feminine, slightly tailored clothes in quality fabrics." She lists Anne Klein, Geoffrey Beene, and Liz Claiborne as her favorite designers. "I don't try to dress younger than I am—I only wear what looks good on me."

Gloria takes great care with her skin but admits that she's not as careful with her fitness regime. "I don't like exercise—I never have. Years ago I

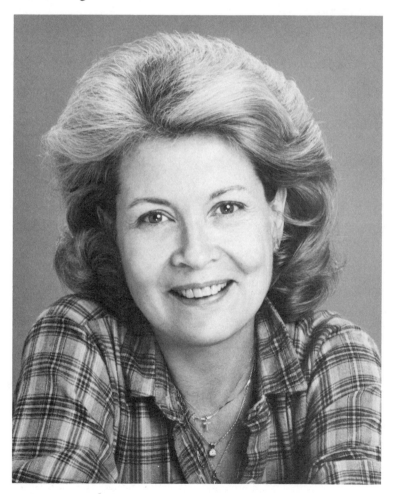

Gloria De Haven

enjoyed dancing, but that was about it. Now I watch my weight constantly. I eat fairly well, but like everyone else, I go on an occasional binge." She doesn't punish herself for her indulgences, however. ("An indulgence is okay now and then—*overindulgence* is what's dangerous," she asserts.)

"The best beauty secret I know," Gloria concludes, "is to like yourself and do the best you can with what you have. You must accept what you are and not wish that you looked like someone else. Instead, make the person that you are better."

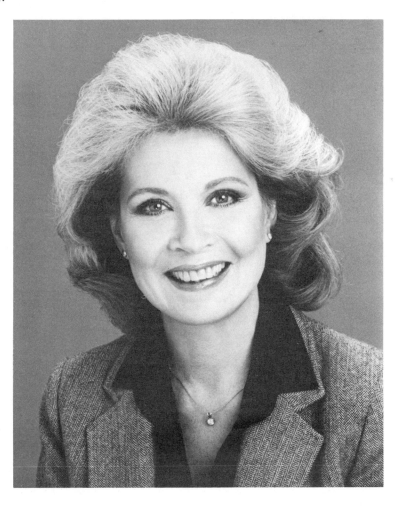

LEONN KALEIKINI

When Leonn Kaleikini graduated from design school and was honored with the America's Next Great Designer award, she was savvy enough to know that she needed to leave her ingenue image behind her. After hair stylist Vanessa Ventura layered Leonn's hair for fullness and added soft shaping with a curling iron, Leonn traded in her leotard for the soft femininity of silk and lace. Her new look is sophisticated yet still accentuates the youthful beauty of her face.

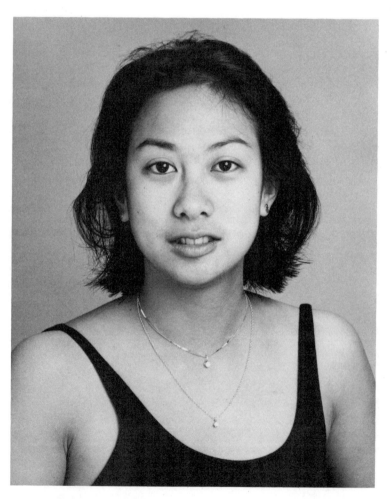

Leonn Kaleikini

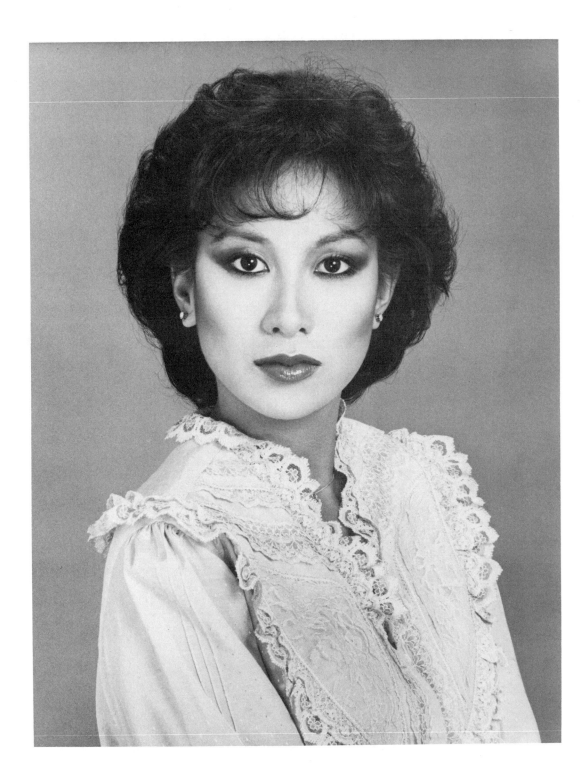

DEIDRE HALL

As Dr. Marlena Evans on "Days of Our Lives," Deidre Hall leads a busy life at a hectic pace. Her wardrobe is casual, devoid of ruffles and frills that complicate her look. Even the pattern of the cardigan sweater she wore for her before picture was too busy for Deidre's tailored personality. A crisp linen blazer worn with her pinstriped blouse simplifies her look and does not detract from her face and fabulous naturally curly hair.

Zora Sloan styled Deidre's thick hair. "I'm lucky that my hair is curly; I don't have to have permanents that might damage it. I have a few highlights put in. I don't even use hot rollers." She washes her hair daily with Nexus shampoo and lets it dry naturally.

As Deidre's before photo indicates, her face is striking without makeup, so she rarely wears any when she's not working. For her after photo, I applied highlighter above her cheekbones, blended up toward the temples, to give her almond-shaped hazel eyes the illusion of an upward slant. Medium brown and dark brown eyebrow pencils were used to fill in her brows, and lip liner, applied outside the natural lines of her somewhat thin lips, gives them a fuller look.

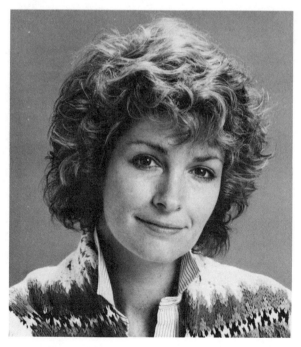

Deidre Hall

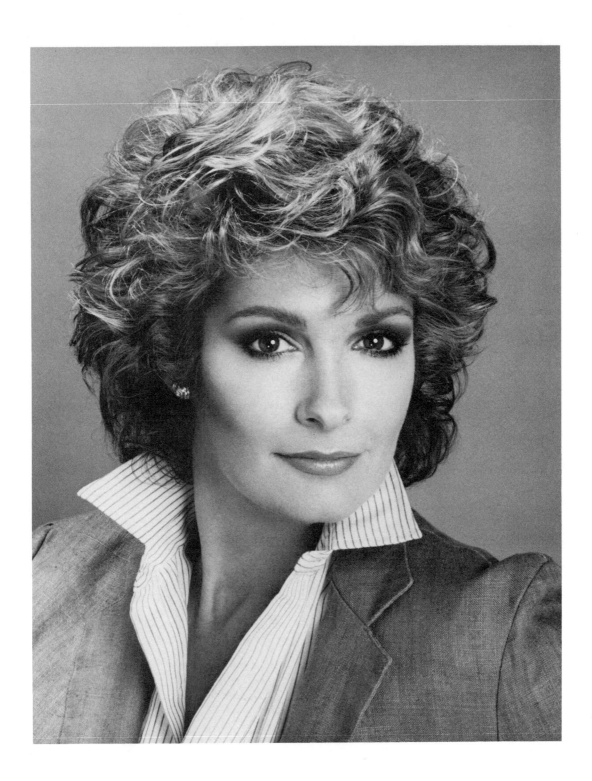

DONNA PESCOW

Pretty, petite Donna Pescow, who played Annette opposite John Travolta in *Saturday Night Fever* and had the title role in the "Angie" TV series, has a round, full face. One simple change makes a major difference in her look—a V-neckline. The geometric line helps elongate her face and draws attention upward. Donna knows the effect of clothes on image, since she literally created her character in *Saturday Night Fever*. "I purposely wore an unflattering sleeveless blouse, cut my nails off, and painted them red—I even intentionally gained weight. Annette was a very different person from the real me." Off screen, Donna loves Calvin Klein's slim-fitting designs.

Hugh Ragan created the perfectly balanced and casual hairstyle that we see in Donna's after photo. She prefers her hair short, which shows off her neck and adds height to her appearance.

I used concealer to hide the discoloration underneath Donna's eyes and a light liquid foundation with pink undertones to balance the sallowness in her face. Heavy accents at her eyes and mouth give her face good proportion.

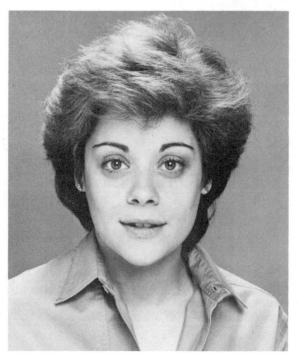

Donna Pescow

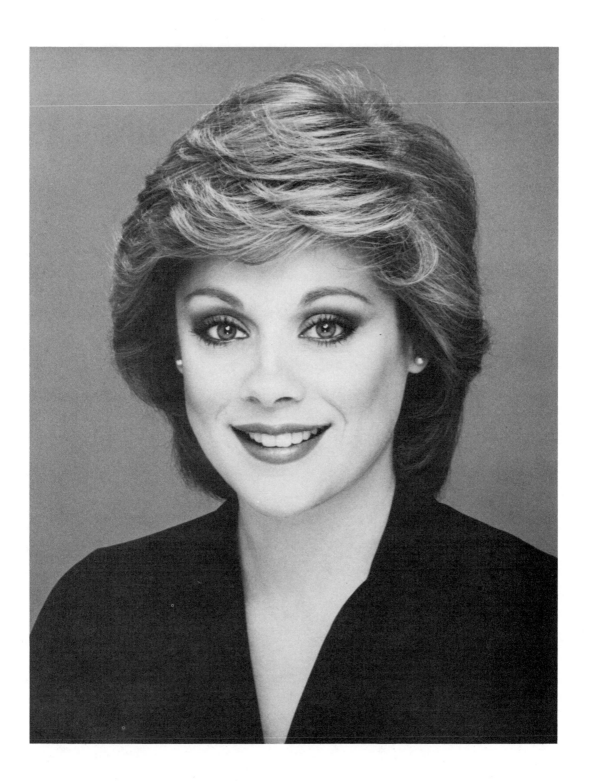

JULIE NEWMAR

Sexy Julie Newmar earned her image playing roles such as Daisy Mae in *L'il Abner,* the sensuous robot in *My Living Doll,* and Cat Woman on TV's "Batman," but she is also truly intelligent, disciplined, and dedicated to her craft.

Every time I see Julie, she is smartly but simply attired in tailored clothes. Her wardrobe is tastefully understated, and she obviously believes that "less is more."

Standing five feet eleven inches, the statuesque beauty never tries to minimize her height. She has perfect posture and carries herself with the self-confidence of the disciplined dancer that she is. She has one of the most beautiful bodies I've ever seen.

Julie has charisma. When I asked her what charisma means to her, she replied, "Energy, energy, energy."

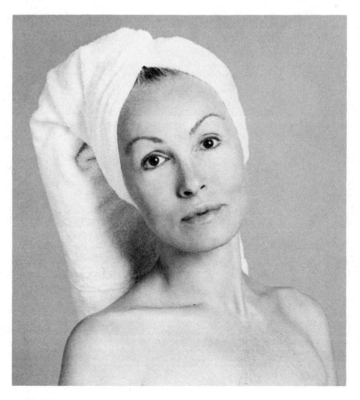

Julie Newmar

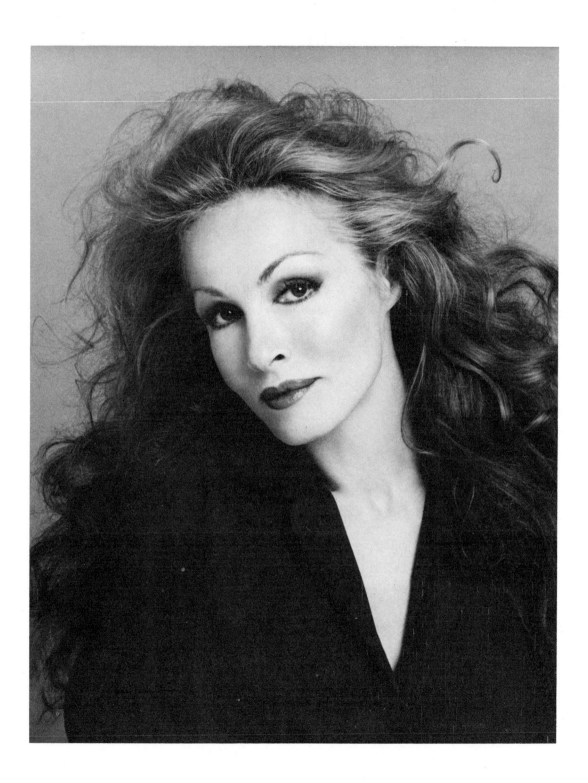

WENDEE WINTERS

When Wendee Winters came to my studio a few years ago, I could tell that she was a very talented actress/comedienne, yet she told me she was having a difficult time with her career. I took an objective look at her: She was pretty, but she had a weight problem. Her nose was relatively large compared to the rest of her features; her hair was mousey; her eyebrows were too dark; and she needed help with her makeup.

Wendee admitted that she wanted to lose weight, so we decided to wait to shoot her photos until she had lost the extra pounds. While she dieted, I suggested she have her hair lightened and restyled. We also lightened her brows two shades. While she was losing weight, I noticed some wonderful changes. Her cheekbones became more prominent and her neck looked longer.

Then I asked if she had ever considered cosmetic surgery to reshape her nose. "Actually, I thought I looked pretty good before," recalls Wendee. "But that was because I never saw my profile. Who sees their profile? I guess I knew I had to do something when people started dropping subtle hints like 'Now that you're a blond, do something about that nose, sweetheart' or 'Get that thing fixed!' At first I was resistant to change, but one day Michael was very frank with me. He asked me if I only wanted to play roles as the funny girl who couldn't get a date. That did it! I made the decision to get my nose done. I chose a doctor who had been highly recommended and had the surgery immediately."

Not long after her total makeover, the new size-5 Wendee returned for her after photo and told me that she had been signed by a leading theatrical agency as well as top commercial agent. Shortly thereafter, she starred in the original cast version of the hit show *Forbidden Broadway* in New York, and she is now enjoying great success with her own cabaret act.

Wendee Winters

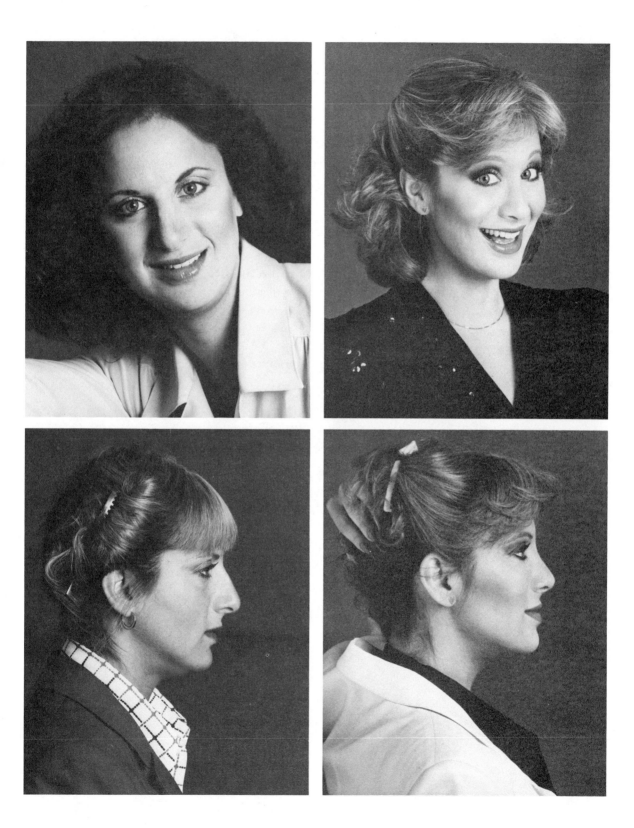

Now available on videocassette!

Michael Maron's Makeover Magic

For ordering information, write or call:

Suntree Video Associates
220 East 23rd Street
Suite 601
New York, NY 10010

(212) 696-1575

INDEX